BUMP AND NOURISH

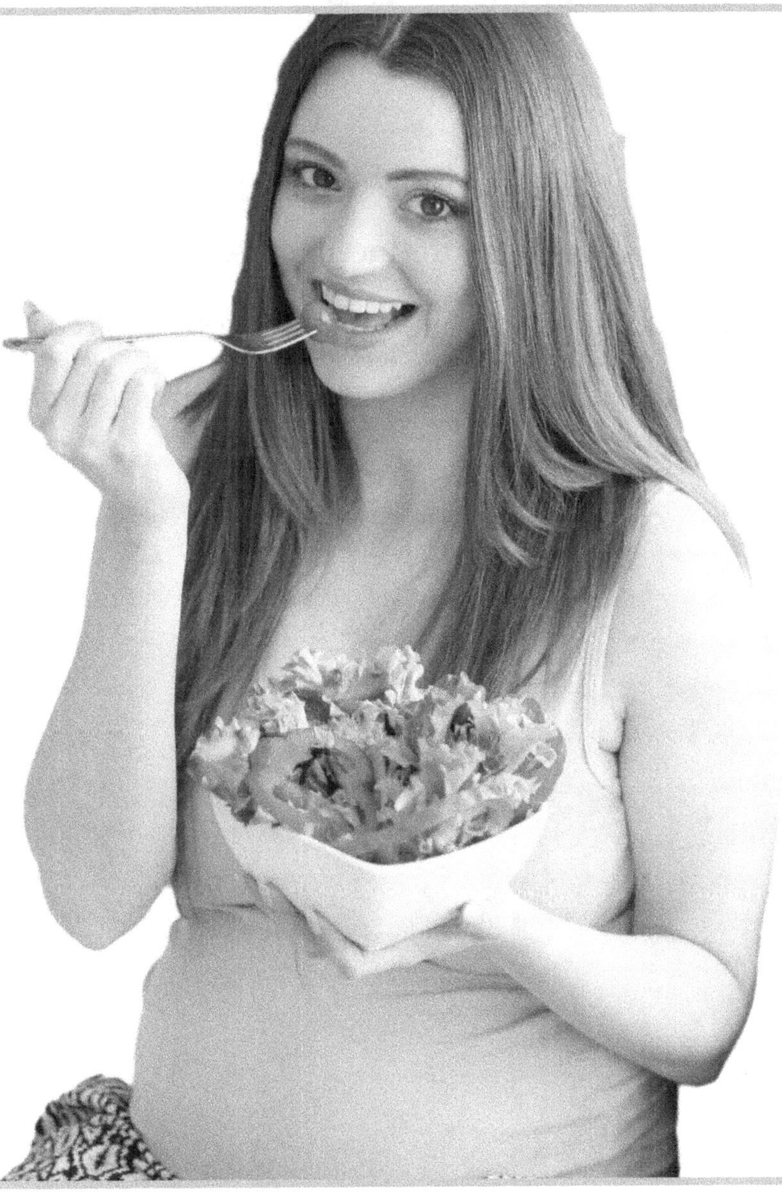

A COLLECTION OF DELICIOUS & HEALTHY RECIPES FOR PREGNANT WOMEN

LUCILLE J. STOKES

COPYRIGHT

DISCLAIMER

The information contained in this book is for general information purposes only. The author makes no representations or warranties of any kind, express or implied, about the completeness, accuracy, reliability, suitability, or availability with respect to the book or the information, products, services, or related graphics contained in the book for any purpose. Any reliance you place on such information is therefore strictly at your own risk. In no event will the author be liable for any loss or damage including without limitation, indirect or consequential loss or damage, or any loss or damage whatsoever arising from loss of data or profits arising out of, or in connection with, the use of this book.

TABLE OF CONTENTS

CHAPTER 1

INTRODUCTION

Importance of healthy eating during pregnancy

As soon as Sarah found out she was pregnant, she was over the moon with excitement. She had longed for this moment for years, planning for every detail to ensure that her baby would have the best start in life possible. However, she had no idea how much the pregnancy would take out of her.

Despite her excitement, the first trimester was a whirlwind of nausea, headaches, and fatigue. Sarah couldn't seem to muster the energy to do anything, let alone cook nutritious meals. The thought of leafy vegetables made her nauseous, and all she could stomach were carbs and sugars.

As time passed, Sarah's lethargy only seemed to increase. She found herself relying more and more on fast food and sugary snacks, convinced that they were the only things that would make her feel better. But despite her best efforts, she kept gaining weight and feeling worse, instead of better.

Sarah's OB/GYN tried to warn her about the dangers of a poor diet during pregnancy and how it could put her and her baby at risk. But Sarah shrugged it off, insisting that she knew what she was doing and that her baby would turn out perfect no matter what. She would worry about losing weight after the baby was born, she told herself.

But when Sarah went into labor, she could tell something was wrong. Her baby's heart rate was low and sluggish, and the doctor immediately had to perform an emergency C-section. When the baby was born, he was small and frail, barely weighing in at 4 pounds. He has immediately whisked away to the NICU, hooked up to machines and tubes.

Sarah was devastated. How could this happen? She had done everything right, or so she thought. The doctor explained that the baby's small size and low birth weight were likely due to her poor diet during pregnancy. The doctor couldn't say for certain that if Sarah had eaten more nutritiously, the baby would have been born at a healthy weight and without any complications, but it's possible.

For days, Sarah watched her tiny, fragile son fight for his life in the NICU. She was wracked with guilt and anxiety, convinced that she had doomed her baby before he even had a chance at life. It was only then that Sarah realized the importance of a healthy pregnancy diet. It wasn't just about ensuring a healthy weight gain and feeling good during pregnancy, it was also about giving her baby the best chance at a healthy start in life.

Sarah vowed to never repeat her mistake again. She spent the next few months researching nutrition and learning how to cook healthy meals that would benefit both her and her baby. She made sure to incorporate plenty of fruits and vegetables, lean proteins, and healthy fats into her diet, all the while monitoring her weight to ensure that she was gaining at a healthy rate.

In the end, Sarah's son pulled through, but with lasting health complications. Sarah was still guilt-ridden, but also determined to make things right. She received the inspiration to compile all her research and trial-and-error efforts in a book to help others who may be in a similar situation as she was. Sarah hopes that her experience serves as a cautionary tale, for all pregnant women to understand the importance and potential consequences of a poor diet during pregnancy.

Maintaining a healthy diet during pregnancy is essential for the mother and the developing fetus. Here are a few reasons why healthy eating is important during pregnancy:

1. Adequate Nutrient Intake: Pregnant women need more nutrients, vitamins, and minerals than non-pregnant women to support fetal development. A well-balanced diet rich in whole grains, fruits, vegetables, lean proteins, and healthy fats can provide the necessary nutrients that nourish the developing fetus and support healthy growth.

2. Lower Risk of Complications: A healthy diet can help reduce the risk of pregnancy complications, such as gestational diabetes, pre-eclampsia, and high blood pressure. Eating properly can also help maintain a healthy weight, which can reduce the risk of complications during labor and delivery.

3. Fetal Development: The quality of nutrients consumed during pregnancy has a significant impact on fetal development, particularly on the development of the brain and nervous system. Healthy eating can help ensure that the fetus receives the proper nutrients for optimal development.

4. Maternal Health: Eating well during pregnancy can help maintain the mother's overall health, including her energy levels, immune function, and mental health. Good nutrition can also aid in postpartum recovery.

Overall, healthy eating during pregnancy is essential for both the mother and the developing fetus. It can reduce the risk of complications, support healthy fetal development, and promote maternal health and well-being.

Common dietary concerns during pregnancy

There are various dietary concerns that pregnant women should be aware of to ensure a healthy pregnancy. Some of the most common concerns include:

1. Nutrient Deficiencies: During pregnancy, certain nutrients are required in greater amounts, and it can be challenging to consume an adequate amount through diet alone. Nutrients such as folic acid, iron, calcium, and Vitamin D, are essential for the growth and development of the fetus. Pregnant women may require supplements to meet their daily needs.

2. Food Safety: Pregnant women are at higher risk of foodborne illnesses such as Listeriosis and Toxoplasmosis. Foods to avoid during pregnancy include unpasteurized dairy products, raw or undercooked meat, and fish containing high levels of mercury such as shark, swordfish, king mackerel, and tilefish.

3. Gestational Diabetes: Some women develop high blood sugar levels during pregnancy, leading to gestational diabetes. A healthy diet low in sugar and refined carbohydrates can help prevent gestational diabetes.

4. Nausea and Vomiting: About 80% of women experience nausea during pregnancy. Choosing small, frequent meals rich in protein, whole grains, fruits, and vegetables, can help alleviate symptoms.

5. Excess Weight Gain: Gaining too much weight during pregnancy can increase the risk of complications like high blood pressure and gestational diabetes. A balanced diet, regular exercise, and monitoring weight gain can help maintain a healthy pregnancy.

6. Digestive Issues: Hormonal changes during pregnancy can lead to constipation. Eating a high-fiber diet with plenty of fluids can help prevent and relieve constipation.

Overall, a nutritious, well-balanced diet, rich in whole foods and minimally processed foods, is crucial during pregnancy. It helps ensure adequate nutrient intake and healthy weight gain while preventing complications for both the mother and the developing fetus.

BREAKFASTS

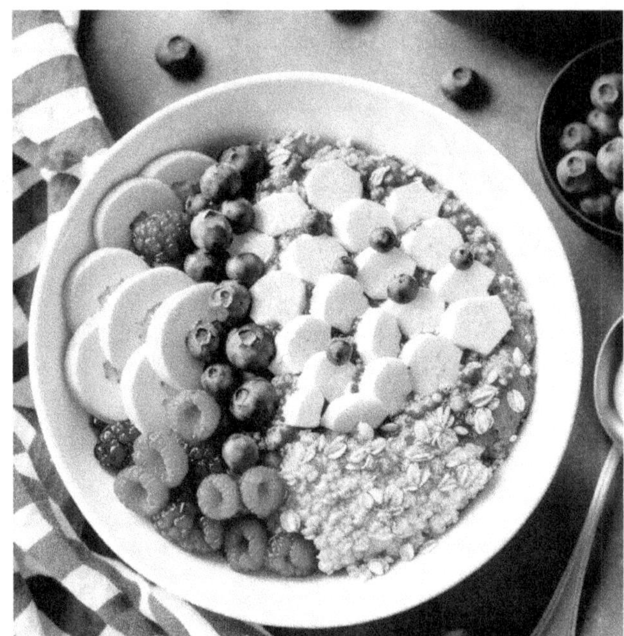

Blueberry Oatmeal Breakfast Bowl is a delicious and nutritious meal that is perfect for starting your day. This meal prep recipe is a great way to make a quick and easy breakfast that is sure to satisfy you. The combination of protein-rich oats, fiber-filled blueberries, and healthy fats from almonds makes it a satisfying breakfast option.

INGREDIENTS:

- 1 cup old-fashioned rolled oats

- 2 cups unsweetened almond milk

- 1 tbsp honey

- 1/2 tsp vanilla extract

- 1/2 tsp ground cinnamon

- 1 cup blueberries

- 1/4 cup slivered almonds

1. In a large saucepan, add the rolled oats, almond milk, honey, vanilla extract, and cinnamon. Stir to combine.

2. Place the saucepan over medium heat and bring the mixture to a boil.

3. Reduce the heat to low and let the mixture simmer for 5-7 minutes, stirring occasionally until the oats are tender and the mixture has thickened.

4. Divide the oatmeal mixture evenly into 4 meal prep containers.

5. Top the oats with blueberries and slivered almonds.

6. Store the meal prep containers in the refrigerator until ready to serve.

Cook Time: 10 minutes

NUTRITIONAL VALUE:

This recipe makes four 1-cup servings. Each serving contains approximately:

Calories: 255 calories; Protein: 8g; Fat: 8g; Carbohydrates: 41g; Fiber: 6g; Sugar: 12g

This Blueberry Oatmeal Breakfast Bowl meal prep is perfect for busy mornings when you don't have time to make breakfast. It can be made ahead of time and stored in the refrigerator, making it an easy grab-and-go option.

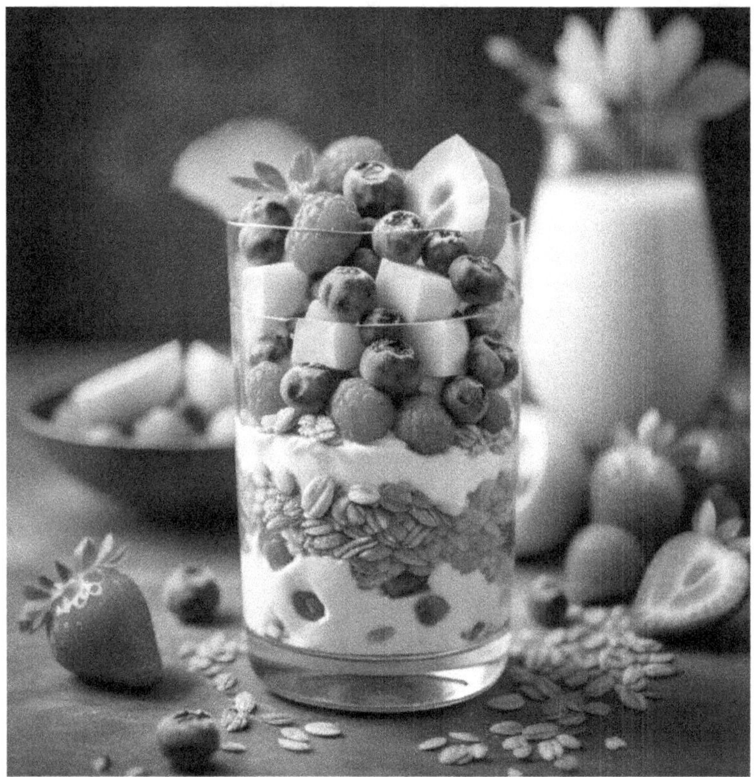

Greek Yogurt Parfait with Fruit and Granola is a delicious and healthy meal prep that is perfect for starting your day or as a mid-day snack. This meal combines the creaminess of Greek yogurt, the sweetness of fresh fruit, and the crunch of granola, making it a satisfying and nutritious option.

INGREDIENTS:

- 2 cups plain Greek yogurt

- 2 cups mixed fresh fruit (e.g. strawberries, blueberries, kiwi, mango)

- 1 cup granola

- 1 tbsp honey

1. Wash and dice the fresh fruit into small pieces.

2. In a bowl, mix together the Greek yogurt and honey until well combined.

3. Divide the yogurt mixture evenly into 4 meal prep containers.

4. Layer the fresh fruit on top of the yogurt mixture.

5. Top each serving with 1/4 cup of granola.

6. Store in the refrigerator until ready to serve.

Cook Time: 10 minutes

NUTRITIONAL VALUE:

This recipe makes four servings. Each serving contains approximately:

Calories: 350 calories; Protein: 19g; Fat: 8g; Carbohydrates: 54g; Fiber: 5g; Sugar: 28g.

Greek Yogurt Parfait with Fruit and Granola is a perfect meal prep option for those who are looking for a healthy and delicious breakfast or snack that can be made ahead of time and stored in the refrigerator. It is rich in protein, fiber, and vitamins, making it a well-balanced meal.

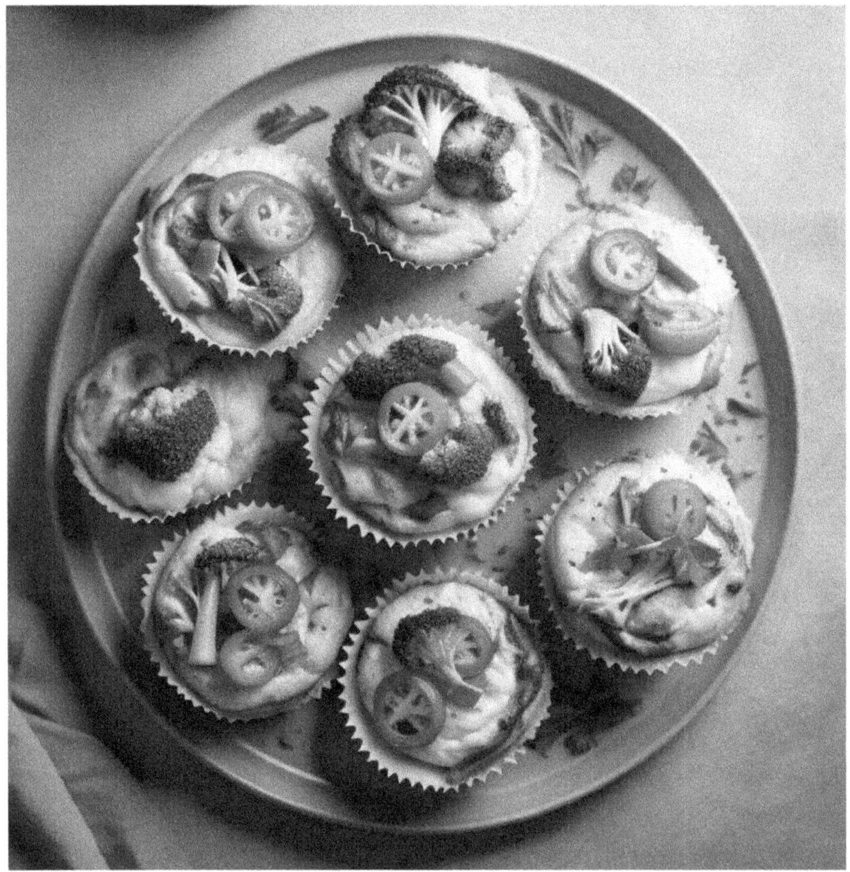

Veggie Packed Egg Muffins are a healthy and delicious meal prep option that is perfect for busy mornings or as a quick snack. These muffins are packed with protein and veggies, making them a nutritious and satisfying option.

INGREDIENTS:

- 6 large eggs

- 1/2 cup milk

- 1 cup mixed veggies, diced (e.g. bell pepper, onion, spinach, mushroom)

- 1/2 cup shredded cheddar cheese

- Salt and pepper, to taste

COOKING INSTRUCTIONS:

1. Preheat the oven to 375°F.

2. In a mixing bowl, whisk together the eggs and milk until well combined.

3. Add in the diced veggies and shredded cheddar cheese, and mix well.

4. Pour the mixture evenly into a muffin tin, filling each cup about 3/4 full.

5. Bake for 20-25 minutes or until the egg muffins are set and golden brown on the top.

6. Let them cool for a few minutes, then remove them from the muffin tin and place them into meal prep containers.

7. Store in the refrigerator until ready to serve.

Cook Time: 25 minutes

NUTRITIONAL VALUE:

This recipe makes six servings. Each serving contains approximately:

Calories: 120 calories; Protein: 9g; Fat: 8g; Carbohydrates: 2g; Fiber: 0.5g; Sugar: 1g.

Veggie Packed Egg Muffins are a great meal prep option for those looking for a healthy and convenient breakfast or snack. The protein and veggies in this meal will help fuel your day, and the delicious taste will keep you satisfied.

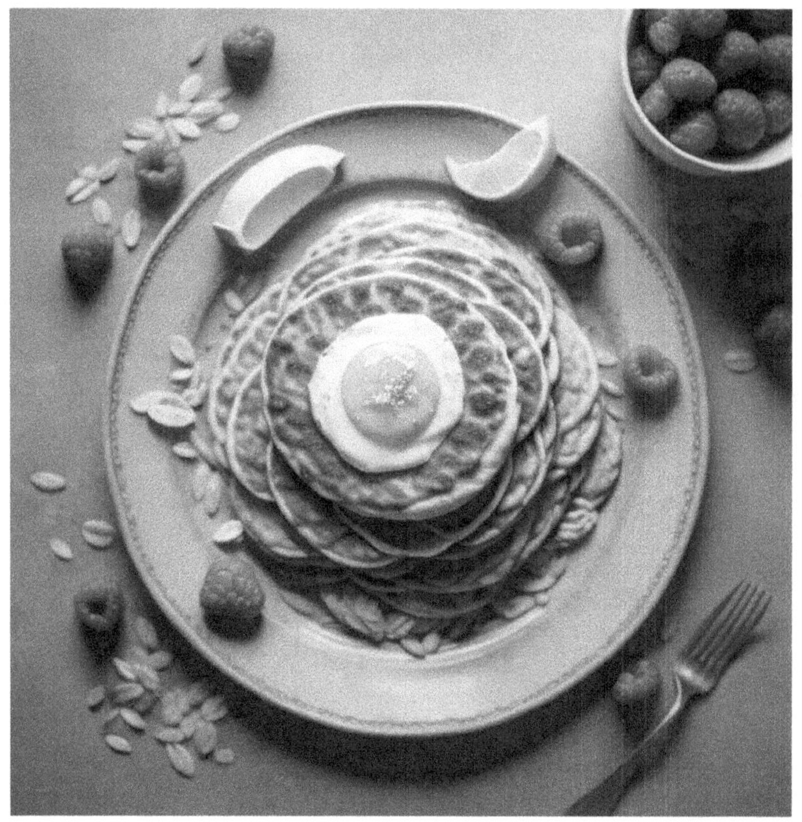

Start your day off with a filling and delicious stack of Banana Oatmeal Pancakes. Made with rolled oats, ripe bananas, and a hint of cinnamon, these pancakes are not only flavor-packed but also full of healthy fiber and complex carbohydrates. Perfect for breakfast, meal prep, or even as a snack, this recipe is easy to make and even easier to enjoy!

INGREDIENTS:

- 2 ripe bananas, mashed

- 2 eggs

- 1/2 cup rolled oats

- 1/2 tsp baking powder

- 1/4 tsp cinnamon

- 1 tsp vanilla extract

- 1 tbsp honey

- Pinch of salt

- Optional toppings: fresh fruit, chopped nuts, maple syrup

COOKING INSTRUCTIONS:

1. In a medium bowl, whisk together mashed bananas and eggs until well combined.

2. Add rolled oats, baking powder, cinnamon, vanilla extract, honey, and salt, and whisk again to combine.

3. Heat a non-stick skillet or griddle over medium heat. Scoop about 1/4 cup of the batter onto the skillet for each pancake.

4. Cook the pancake for about 2-3 minutes, then flip and cook for another 2-3 minutes until both sides are golden brown.

5. Repeat with remaining batter, making sure to spray the skillet with cooking spray between each batch.

6. Let the pancakes cool before storing them in an airtight container in the fridge. Reheat by microwaving for 30-40 seconds before serving.

Cook Time: 15-20 minutes

NUTRITIONAL VALUE (per serving, makes 8 small pancakes):

Calories: 69; Fat: 1.5g; Carbohydrates: 12.5g; Fiber: 1.5g; Sugar: 5.5g; Protein: 2.5g.

These Banana Oatmeal Pancakes are a great way to start your day, and can even be enjoyed as a mid-day snack. The recipe is easy to make, and it's packed with fiber, protein, and complex carbs to keep you satisfied and energized all morning long. Try them out this week and enjoy the delicious taste of homemade pancakes!

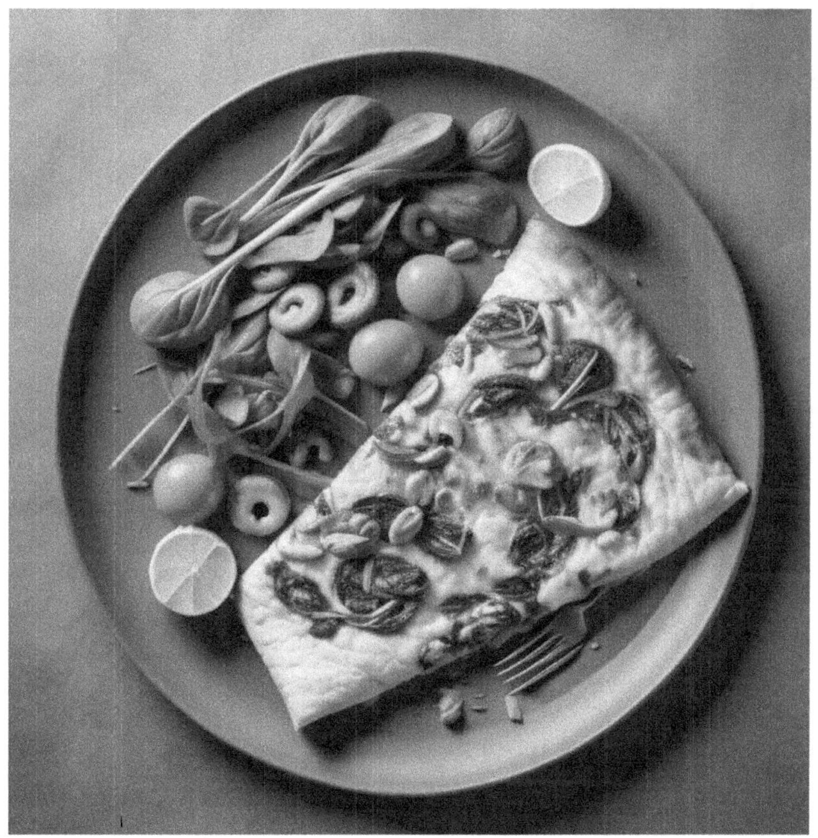

Looking for a delicious and nutritious breakfast option? This Spinach and Mushroom Omelet Meal Prep recipe is a surefire way to start your day off right. Made with fluffy eggs, sautéed spinach, and mushrooms, this dish is packed with protein, fiber, and vitamins. Plus, it's easy to make and perfect for meal prep!

INGREDIENTS:

- 4 eggs

- 1 cup fresh spinach, chopped

- 1 cup mushrooms, sliced

- 1/4 cup onion, chopped

- 1 clove garlic, minced

- Salt and pepper to taste

- Cooking spray

- Optional toppings: diced tomatoes, shredded cheese, avocado

COOKING INSTRUCTIONS:

1. In a medium bowl, whisk together the eggs until light and frothy. Set aside.

2. In a skillet over medium-high heat, spray the cooking spray, then sauté the chopped onion and garlic until onions are translucent.

3. Add the chopped spinach and sliced mushrooms to the skillet and cook for 3-5 minutes until the vegetables are tender.

4. Reduce heat to medium, pour the whisked eggs over the vegetable mixture, allowing the eggs to cook for approximately 2-3 minutes.

5. Once the eggs begin to set, use a spatula to gently fold the omelet in half.

6. Cook the omelet for another 2-3 minutes until the eggs are set.

7. Let the omelet cool, then slice into 4 equal servings.

8. Store in an airtight container in the fridge for up to 3-4 days.

Cook Time: 15-20 minutes

NUTRITIONAL VALUE (per serving):

Calories: 110; Fat: 5g; Carbohydrates: 4g; Fiber: 1g; Sugar: 2.5g; Protein: 10g.

This Spinach and Mushroom Omelet Meal Prep recipe is easy to make and packed with nutrients to keep you full and satisfied all day long. It's a great option for a healthy breakfast or brunch, and can even be enjoyed as a midday snack. Give it a try and enjoy the rich flavor and nourishing benefits of this tasty omelet!

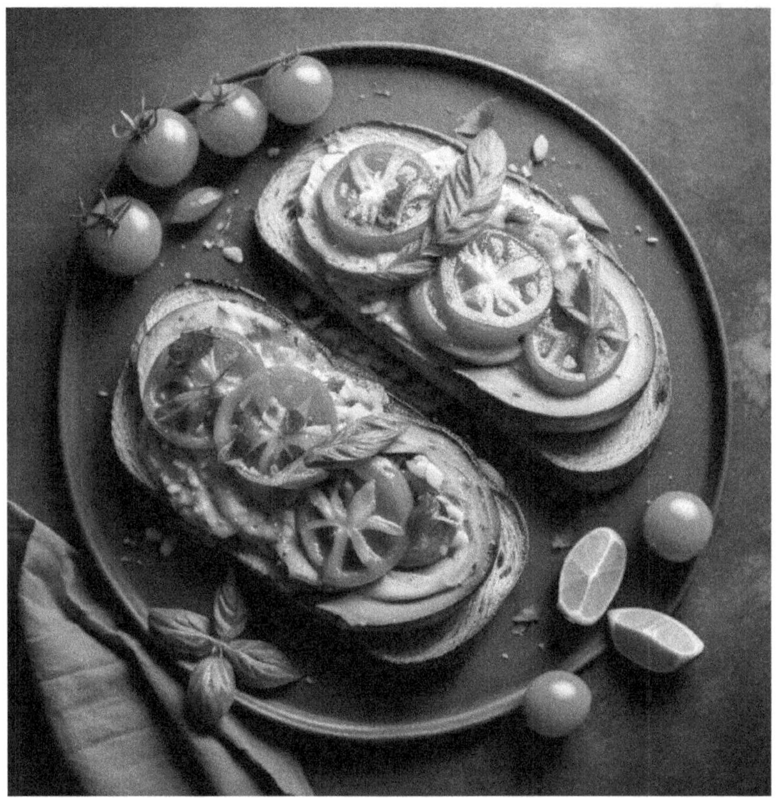

If you're looking for a quick and easy breakfast or snack option, this Grilled Avocado and Tomato Toast Meal Prep recipe is the way to go. Made with ceamy avocado, juicy tomatoes, and hearty whole-grain bread, this dish is packed with healthy fats, fiber, and protein. Plus, it's easy to make and perfect for busy mornings!

INGREDIENTS:

- 1 ripe avocado, sliced

- 1 medium tomato, sliced

- 2 slices whole-grain bread

- 1 tbsp olive oil

- Salt and pepper to taste

- Optional toppings: crumbled feta cheese, chopped fresh herbs (such as parsley or basil)

Cooking Instructions:

1. Preheat a grill pan or skillet over medium-high heat.

2. Brush the sliced avocado and tomato with olive oil and season with salt and pepper.

3. Place the avocado and tomato slices on the grill pan or skillet, and grill for 1-2 minutes on each side or until they are slightly charred.

4. Toast the slices of bread.

5. Top each slice of toast with the grilled avocado and tomato slices.

6. Add toppings of your choice, such as crumbled feta cheese or chopped fresh herbs.

7. Let the toast cool, then store in an airtight container in the fridge for up to 2 days.

Cook Time: 10-15 minutes

NUTRITIONAL VALUE (per serving):

Calories: 270; Fat: 19g; Carbohydrates: 20g; Fiber: 9g; Sugar: 3g; Protein: 6g.

This Grilled Avocado and Tomato Toast Meal Prep recipe is a perfect way to start your day or fuel up with a snack. It's easy to make, packed with healthy ingredients, and can be made ahead of time for busy mornings. Give it a try and savor the delicious flavors and benefits of this wholesome dish!

7. BLUEBERRY OAT MUFFINS

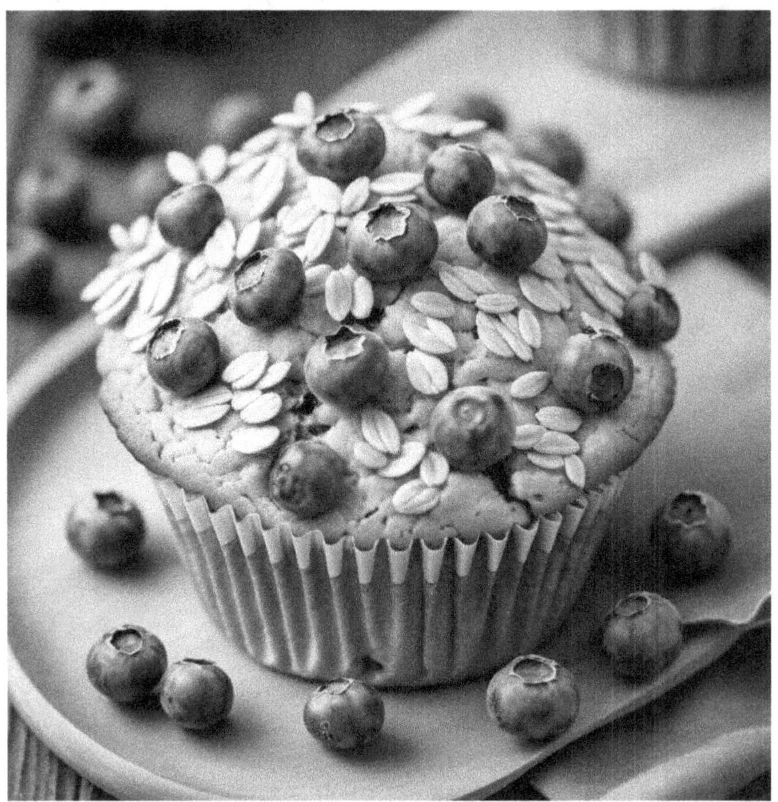

Start your day off on a sweet and wholesome note with these Blueberry Oat Muffins. Made with fresh juicy blueberries, hearty oats, and a touch of honey, these muffins are a delicious and nourishing breakfast or snack option. Plus, they're easy to make and perfect for meal prep!

INGREDIENTS:

- 1 1/2 cups rolled oats

- 1 cup all-purpose flour

- 1/4 cup honey

- 1/4 cup unsweetened applesauce

- 2 ripe bananas, mashed

- 1 tsp baking powder

- 1/2 tsp baking soda

- 1/2 tsp salt

- 1/4 cup almond milk

- 1 egg

- 1 tsp vanilla extract

- 1 cup fresh blueberries

COOKING INSTRUCTIONS:

1. Preheat the oven to 350°F and line a muffin tin with 12 muffin liners.

2. In a large mixing bowl, combine the rolled oats, flour, baking powder, baking soda, and salt.

3. In a separate mixing bowl, whisk together the egg, honey, applesauce, mashed bananas, almond milk, and vanilla extract.

4. Pour the wet ingredients into the dry ingredients and stir until well combined.

5. Fold in the fresh blueberries.

6. Use a spoon to distribute the batter evenly among the muffin cups.

7. Bake for 20-25 minutes, or until a toothpick inserted into the center of a muffin comes out clean.

8. Let the muffins cool, then store in an airtight container in the fridge for up to 5 days.

Cook Time: 20-25 minutes

NUTRITIONAL VALUE (per muffin):

Calories: 130; Fat: 1.5g; Carbohydrates: 28g; Fiber: 2.5g; Sugar: 11g; Protein: 3.5g.

These Blueberry Oat Muffins are a delicious and healthy breakfast or snack option that are perfect for meal prep. They're easy to make, packed with fiber and nutrients, and can be enjoyed throughout the week. Give this recipe a try and enjoy the sweet and rich flavor of these muffins.

CHAPTER 3

SNACKS

1. APPLE SLICES WITH ALMOND BUTTER

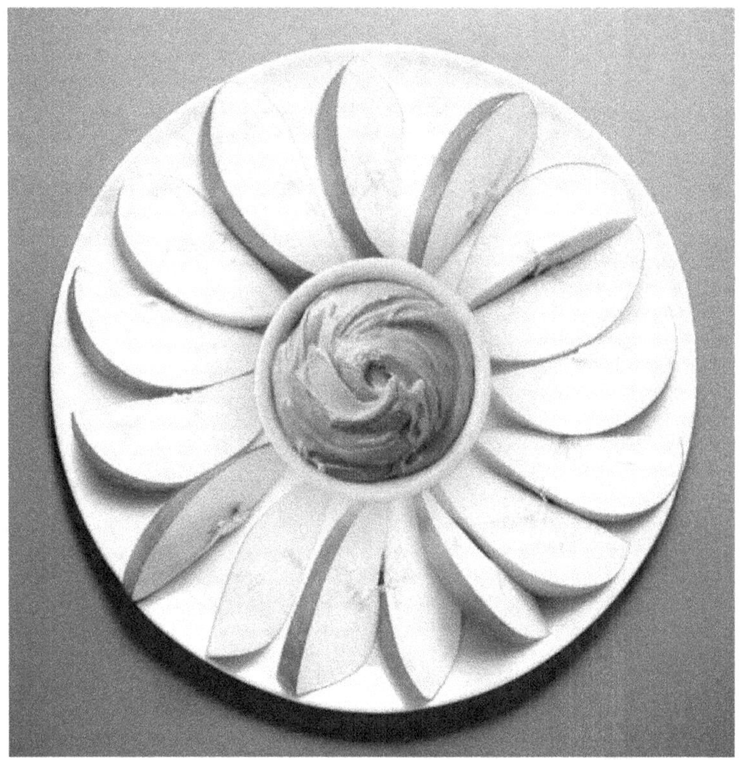

Apple slices with almond butter make a tasty and nutritious snack that will give you energy without causing a crash. This simple yet delicious recipe takes only minutes to make and is perfect for those times when you need a quick boost during the day.

INGREDIENTS:

- 2 apples (Honeycrisp, Gala, or Granny Smith)

- 1/4 cup almond butter

- 2 teaspoons honey

- 1/2 teaspoon cinnamon

COOKING INSTRUCTIONS:

1. Wash the apples and slice them into thin wedges.

2. In a small bowl, mix together the almond butter, honey, and cinnamon until well combined.

3. Serve the apple wedges with a dollop of almond butter mixture on each slice.

Cook Time: 5 minutes

NUTRITIONAL VALUE:

This recipe makes four servings. Each serving (about six apple wedges with almond butter) contains approximately:

- Calories: 160 calories

Protein: 4g; Fat: 10g; Carbohydrates: 16g; Fiber: 4g; Sugar: 11g.

Apple slices with almond butter is a healthy snack that provides a balance of healthy fats, carbohydrates, and protein. The sweetness of the apples combined with the nutty flavor of the almond butter creates a satisfying and nutritious snack that will keep you full and satisfied.

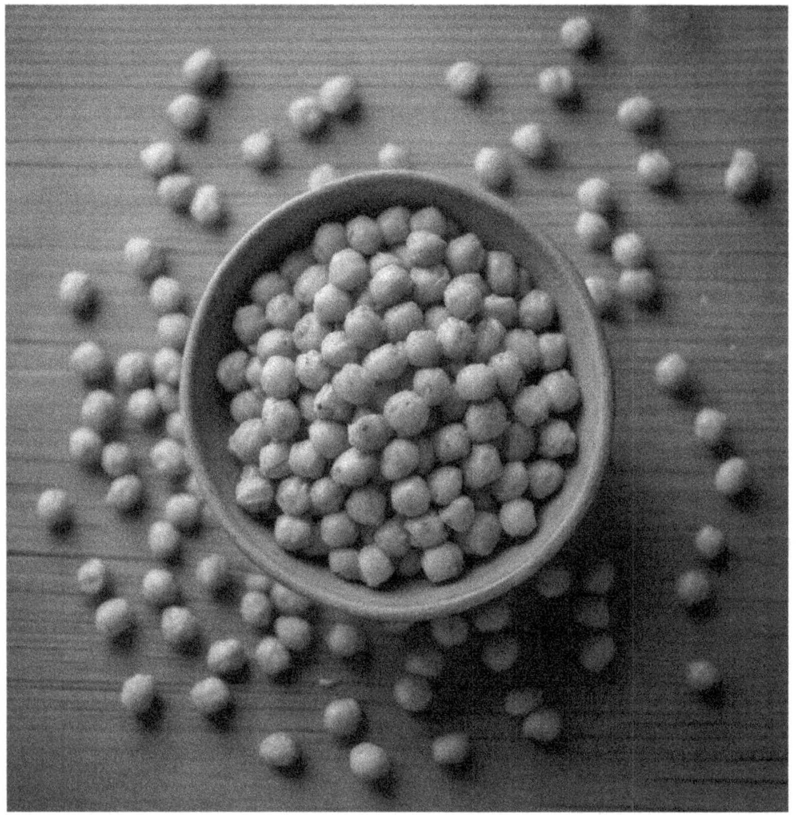

Roasted chickpeas are a delicious and nutritious snack that is perfect for vegans, gluten-free eaters, and anyone who is looking for a healthy alternative to chips or crackers. They are crispy, crunchy, and packed with protein and fiber, making them a satisfying and filling snack.

INGREDIENTS:

- 1 can chickpeas (15 oz)

- 1 tablespoon olive oil

- 1/2 teaspoon salt

- 1/2 teaspoon garlic powder

- 1/2 teaspoon smoked paprika

1. Preheat the oven to 400°F.

2. Drain and rinse the chickpeas, then pat them dry with a paper towel.

3. In a small mixing bowl, combine the olive oil, salt, garlic powder, and smoked paprika.

4. Add the chickpeas to the bowl and toss well to coat.

5. Spread the chickpeas in a single layer on a baking sheet lined with parchment paper.

6. Bake for 20-30 minutes, until chickpeas are crispy and golden brown.

7. Remove from the oven and let cool for 5 minutes.

8. Serve and enjoy.

Cook Time: 20-30 minutes

Nutritional Value: This recipe makes four servings.

Each serving (about 1/4 cup) contains approximately:

Calories: 120 calories; Protein: 6g; Fat: 4g; Carbohydrates: 16g; Fiber: 4g; Sugar: 1g.

Roasted chickpeas are a healthy and delicious snack that is perfect for any time of day. They are high in fiber and protein, making them a great choice for keeping you feeling full and satisfied between meals. Try different flavor combinations, such as chili powder or cumin, to create your own unique and flavorful snack.

3. SMOOTHIE BOWL WITH BERRIES AND SEEDS

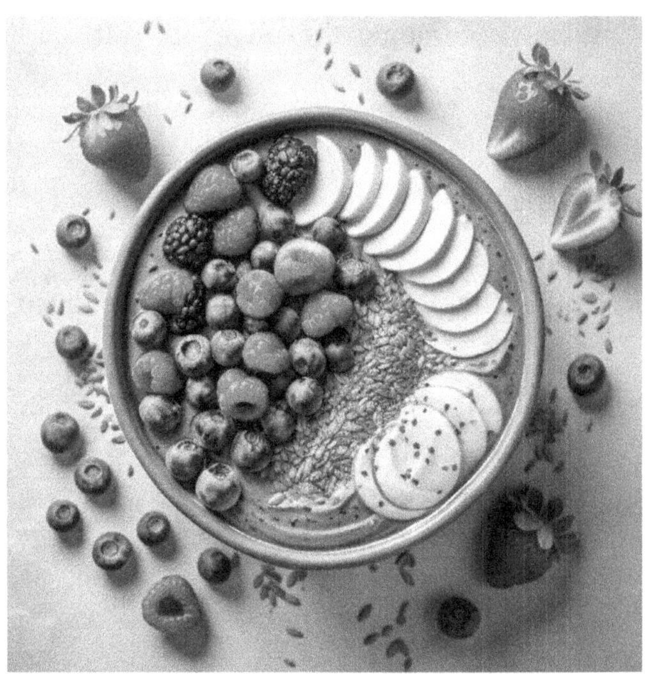

A smoothie bowl is a nutritious and refreshing snack that can be customized with your favorite fruits, seeds, and toppings. This particular recipe features a delicious blend of berries and seeds for a tasty and nutritious snack that is perfect for any time of day.

INGREDIENTS:

- 1 cup frozen mixed berries

- 1/2 cup vanilla Greek yogurt (or dairy-free yogurt)

- 1/4 cup almond milk (or any other milk you prefer)

- 1 tablespoon chia seeds

- 1 tablespoon flax seeds

- Toppings of your choice (such as sliced banana, granola, or nuts)

COOKING INSTRUCTIONS:

1. In a blender, combine the frozen berries, Greek yogurt, and almond milk.

2. Blend until smooth and creamy.

3. Pour the smoothie into a bowl.

4. Sprinkle chia seeds and flax seeds over the top of the smoothie bowl.

5. Add your favorite toppings, such as sliced banana, granola, or nuts.

6. Serve immediately.

Cook Time: 5 minutes

NUTRITIONAL VALUE:

This recipe makes one serving. Each serving contains approximately:

Calories: 270 calories; Protein: 17g; Fat: 11g; Carbohydrates: 30g; Fiber: 10g; Sugar: 16g.

Smoothie bowls are a delicious and nutritious snack that is perfect for those times when you need a quick and healthy pick-me-up. This recipe is packed with protein, fiber, and healthy fats, making it a satisfying snack that will keep you full and energized for hours. Plus, the berries provide a ton of antioxidants and vitamins for an extra boost of nutrition.

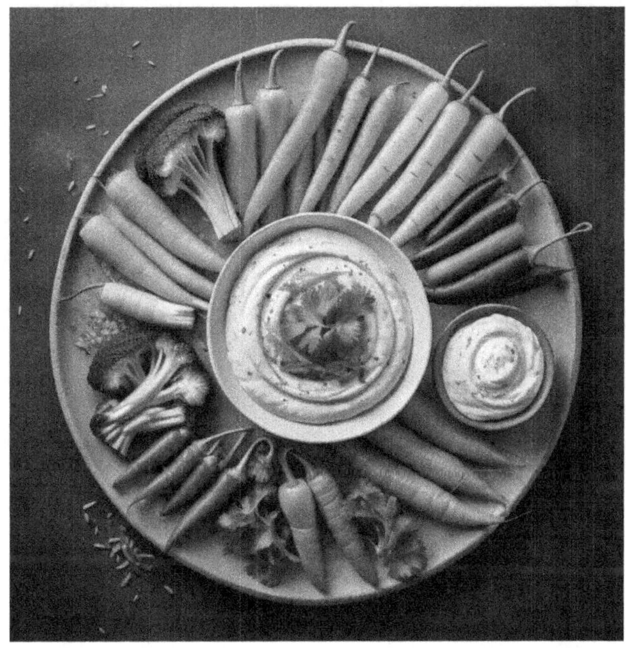

Looking for a healthy and delicious snack option? Look no further than Veggie Sticks and Hummus! Made with colorful bell peppers, crunchy carrots, and creamy hummus, this snack is packed with fiber, vitamins, and healthy fats. Plus, it's easy to make and perfect for meal prep!

INGREDIENTS:

- 3 bell peppers (1 red, 1 yellow, 1 green)

- 4 carrots

- 1 container of hummus (10 oz)

COOKING INSTRUCTIONS:

1. Wash the bell peppers and carrots and dry with a clean kitchen towel.

2. Slice the bell peppers into thin strips and cut the carrots into sticks.

3. Divide the veggie sticks into individual meal prep containers or ziplock bags.

4. Add a dollop of hummus to each container or bag.

5. Seal the containers or bags and store in the fridge for up to 5 days.

Prep Time: 10 minutes

NUTRITIONAL VALUE **(per serving):**

Calories: 120; Fat: 7g; Carbohydrates: 13g; Fiber: 5g; Sugar: 6g; Protein: 4g.

This Veggie Sticks and Hummus Meal Prep is perfect for a quick and healthy snack on-the-go. It's packed with colorful veggies, healthy fats, and protein, making it the perfect combination to fuel your body between meals. Give this recipe a try and enjoy the fresh and delicious taste of raw veggies paired with creamy hummus.

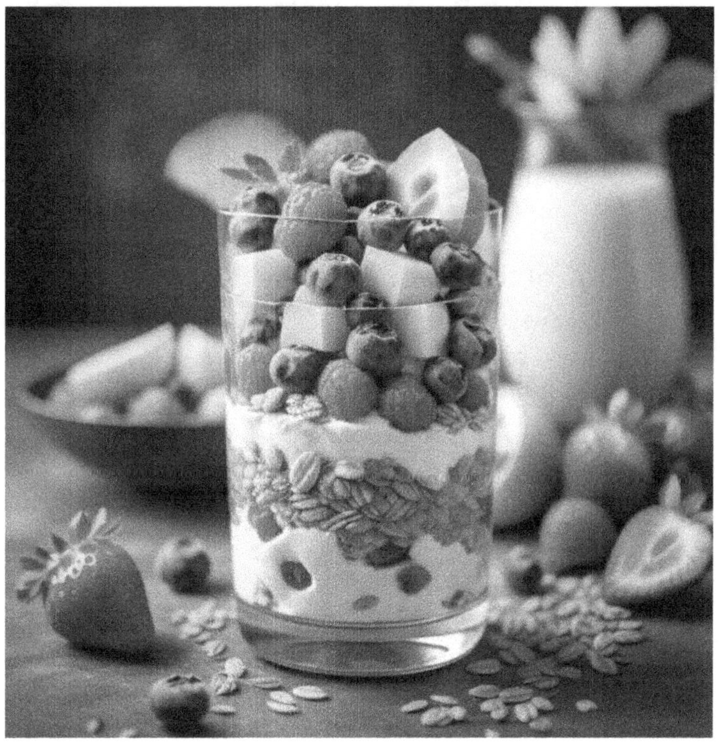

Looking for a sweet and satisfying snack option? Try this Greek Yogurt Parfait! Made with creamy Greek yogurt, juicy berries, and crunchy granola, it's a perfect combination of protein, fiber, and healthy fats. Plus, it's easy to make and perfect for meal prep!

INGREDIENTS:

- 2 cups plain Greek yogurt

- 1 cup mixed berries (such as strawberries, blueberries, raspberries)

- 1/2 cup granola

- 1 tbsp honey

COOKING INSTRUCTIONS:

1. Wash the berries and dry with a clean kitchen towel. Cut the strawberries into small pieces.

2. In a small bowl, mix together the Greek yogurt and honey.

3. Divide the honey yogurt mixture into individual meal prep containers.

4. Layer the berries on top of the yogurt mixture.

5. Sprinkle the granola on top of the berries.

6. Seal the containers and store in the fridge for up to 3 days.

Prep Time: 10 minutes

NUTRITIONAL VALUE **(per serving):**

Calories: 260; Fat: 5g; Carbohydrates: 44g; Fiber: 5g; Sugar: 25g; Protein: 16g.

This Greek Yogurt Parfait Meal Prep is a delicious and healthy snack option that's perfect for satisfying your sweet tooth. It's a great source of protein, fiber, and healthy fats, making it the perfect snack to keep you feeling full and satisfied between meals. Give this recipe a try and enjoy the sweet and creamy taste of Greek yogurt paired with juicy berries and crunchy granola.

6. ENERGY BALLS MEAL

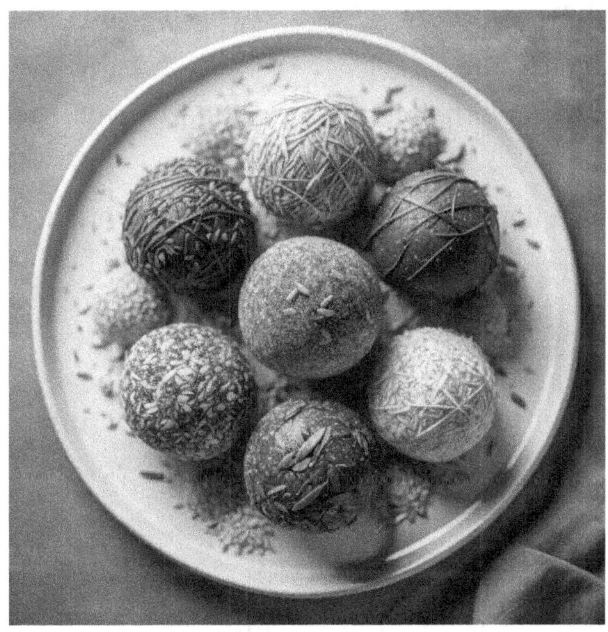

Looking for a quick and healthy snack option that's energizing and delicious? Try these Energy Balls! Made with wholesome ingredients like oats, nut butter, and honey, these Energy Balls are packed with protein, fiber, healthy fats, and natural sweetness. Plus, they're easy to make and perfect for meal prep!

INGREDIENTS:

- 1 cup rolled oats

- 1/2 cup nut butter (such as almond, peanut, or cashew)

- 1/4 cup honey

- 1/4 cup chia seeds

- 1/4 cup shredded coconut (unsweetened)

- 1 tsp vanilla extract

COOKING INSTRUCTIONS:

1. In a large mixing bowl, combine all ingredients and mix well.

2. Use a tablespoon to scoop the mixture and roll into small balls.

3. Place the balls on a baking sheet lined with parchment paper.

4. Freeze the balls for 15-20 minutes or until firm.

5. Store the balls in an airtight container in the fridge for up to 2 weeks.

Prep Time: 20 minutes

NUTRITIONAL VALUE **(per serving - 2 balls):**

Calories: 180; Fat: 10g; Carbohydrates: 19g; Fiber: 5g; Sugar: 7g; Protein: 6g.

These Energy Balls are a delicious and healthy snack option that's perfect for boosting your energy levels throughout the day. They're packed with protein, fiber, healthy fats, and natural sweetness, making them a great alternative to processed snacks. Give this recipe a try and enjoy the tasty and nutritious benefits of these Energy Balls.

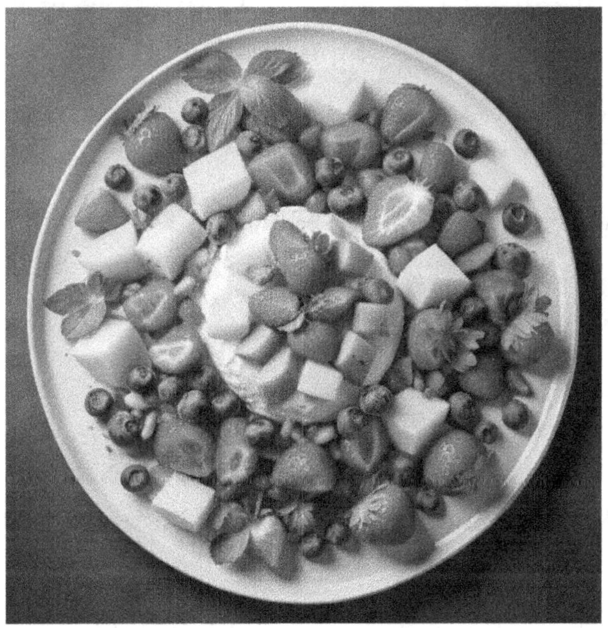

Looking for a healthy and refreshing snack option during pregnancy? Try this Fruit Salad! Made with a variety of colorful fruits, it's packed with vitamins, minerals, and antioxidants that are essential for your growing baby. Plus, it's easy to make and perfect for meal prep!

INGREDIENTS:

- 2 cups chopped fresh fruit (such as strawberries, blueberries, kiwi, mango, pineapple, and grapes)

- 1/2 lime, juiced

- 1 tbsp honey

COOKING INSTRUCTIONS:

1. Chop the fruits into bite-sized pieces and mix them together in a large bowl.

2. In a small bowl, mix together the lime juice and honey until well combined.

3. Pour the lime-honey dressing over the fruit and mix well.

4. Divide the fruit salad into individual meal prep containers.

5. Seal the containers and store in the fridge for up to 3 days.

Prep Time: 10 minutes

NUTRITIONAL VALUE **(per serving):**

Calories: 100; Fat: 0g; Carbohydrates: 26g; Fiber: 3g; Sugar: 20g; Protein: 1g.

This Fruit Salad Meal Prep is a delicious and nutritious snack option that's perfect for pregnancy. It's packed with vitamins, minerals, and antioxidants that are important for your baby's development, and it's easy to make and store for later. Give this recipe a try and enjoy the sweet and refreshing taste of fresh fruits!

LUNCHES

1. QUINOA AND ROASTED VEGETABLE SALAD

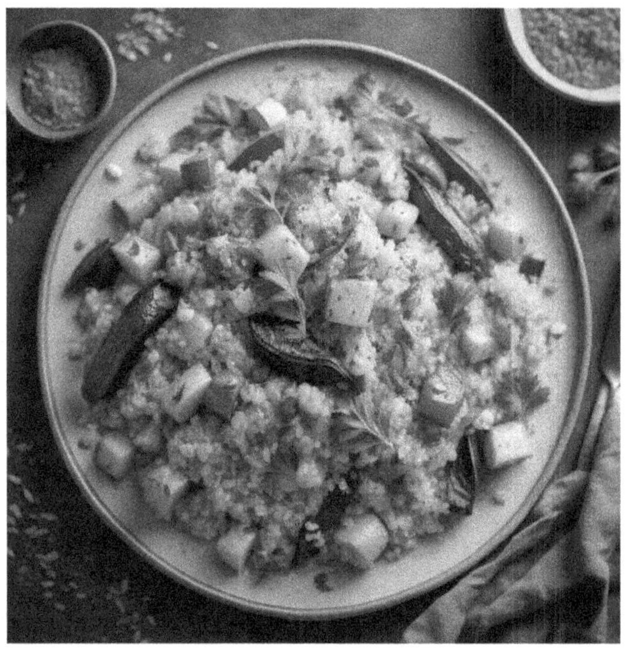

Quinoa and Roasted Vegetable Salad is a healthy and flavorful meal prep that is perfect for lunch or dinner. This salad is packed with protein and veggies, making it a nutritious and satisfying option.

INGREDIENTS:

- 1 cup quinoa

- 2 cups water or vegetable broth

- 2 cups mixed vegetables, diced (e.g. bell pepper, zucchini, onion, mushroom)

- 2 cloves garlic, minced

- 1 tablespoon olive oil

- Salt and pepper, to taste

- 1/4 cup crumbled feta cheese (optional)

1. Preheat the oven to 400°F.

2. Rinse quinoa in a fine mesh strainer and place in a pot with the water or broth. Bring to a boil, then lower heat and simmer for 15-20 minutes or until the quinoa is fluffy and the liquid has been absorbed.

3. In a bowl, mix the diced vegetables, minced garlic, olive oil, salt and pepper until vegetables are coated.

4. Spread out the vegetables onto a baking sheet in a single layer and roast for 20-25 minutes, or until tender and slightly golden.

5. Once the quinoa and vegetables are cooked, mix together in a large bowl.

6. Store in meal prep containers, and sprinkle feta cheese on top (optional).

7. Serve chilled or reheat in the microwave when ready to eat.

Cook Time: 45 minutes

NUTRITIONAL VALUE:

This recipe makes four servings. Each serving contains approximately:

Calories: 320 calories; Protein: 11g; Fat: 9g; Carbohydrates: 50g; Fiber: 7g; Sugar: 5g.

Quinoa and Roasted Vegetable Salad is a delicious and healthy meal prep option that is perfect for lunch or dinner. The protein and veggies in this meal will provide you with the nutrients and energy you need to get through your day, while the delicious taste will keep you satisfied.

2. SWEET POTATO AND BLACK BEAN TACOS

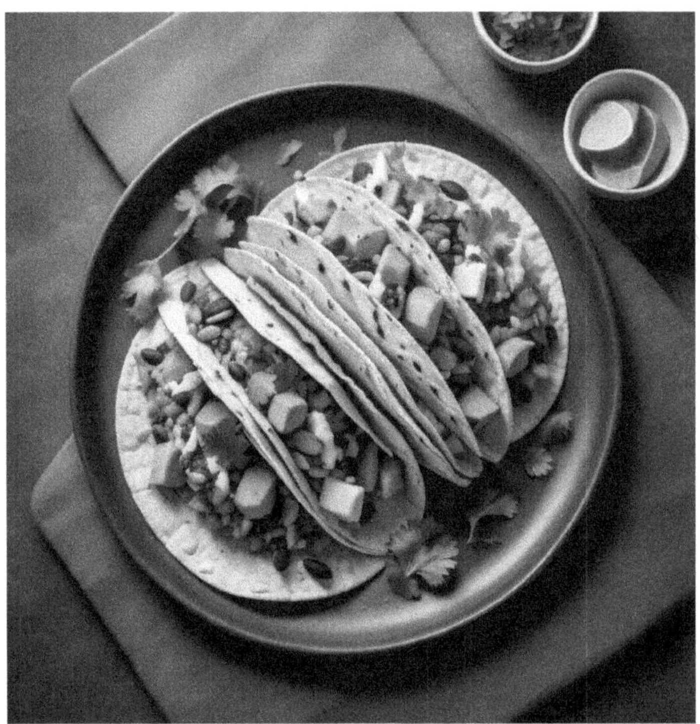

Sweet Potato and Black Bean Tacos are a delicious and healthy meal prep that is perfect for lunch or dinner. These tacos are flavorful and packed with protein and veggies, making them a nutritious and satisfying option.

INGREDIENTS:

- 2 large sweet potatoes, peeled and diced

- 1 can black beans, rinsed and drained

- 1 red onion, diced

- 2 cloves garlic, minced

- 1 tablespoon olive oil

- 2 teaspoons chili powder

- 1 teaspoon ground cumin

- Salt and pepper, to taste

- Corn tortillas

- Optional toppings: avocado, salsa, cilantro

COOKING INSTRUCTIONS:

1. Preheat the oven to 400°F.

2. Peel and cut sweet potatoes into small pieces.

3. In a bowl mix sweet potatoes, diced red onion, minced garlic, olive oil, chili powder, ground cumin, salt and pepper until everything is well coated.

4. Spread the sweet potato mix out onto a lined baking sheet. Bake for 20-30 minutes or until sweet potatoes are soft and caramelized.

5. While the sweet potatoes are baking, rinse the black beans and heat them in a saucepan on medium heat for 5-10 minutes.

6. Once the sweet potatoes and black beans are done, heat the corn tortillas in a pan.

7. Assemble tacos with sweet potatoes and black beans, and add desired toppings (optional).

8. Store in meal prep containers.

Cook Time: 45 minutes

This recipe makes four servings. Each serving contains approximately:

Calories: 360 calories; Protein: 13g; Fat: 7g; Carbohydrates: 64g; Fiber: 14g; Sugar: 10g.

Sweet Potato and Black Bean Tacos are a delicious and healthy meal prep option that is perfect for lunch or dinner. The combination of sweet potatoes and black beans provides a variety of nutrients and plant-based protein to keep you feeling full and satisfied. The flavorful toppings like avocado and salsa also provide added nutrition and taste.

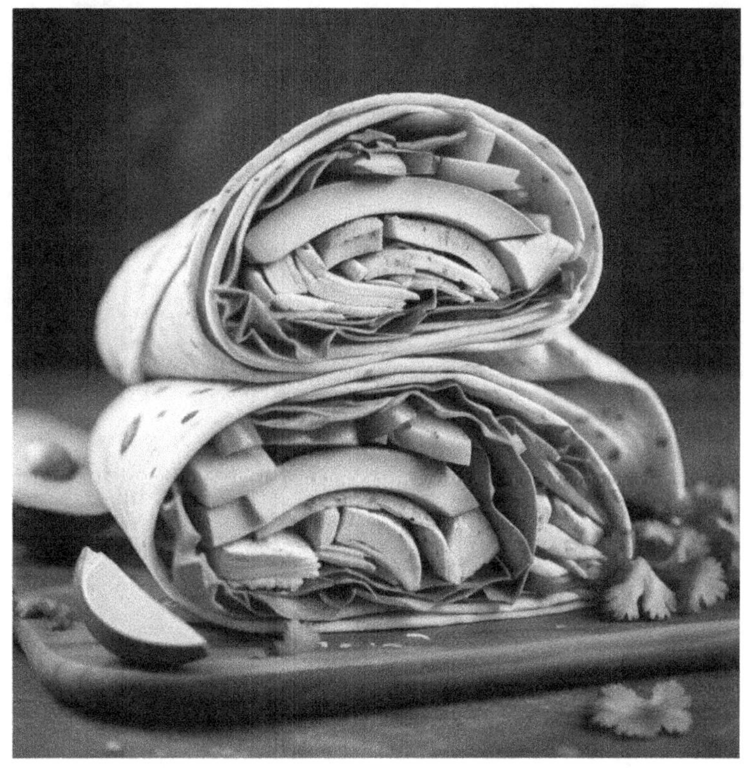

Turkey and Avocado Wrap is a tasty and nutritious meal prep that is perfect for lunch. This wrap is packed with protein and healthy fats, making it a satisfying and filling option.

INGREDIENTS:

- 4 whole wheat tortillas

- 8 oz. sliced turkey breast

- 1 avocado, sliced

- 1 bell pepper, sliced

- 1 small red onion, sliced

- 2 tablespoons hummus (or other spread of your choice)

- Salt and pepper, to taste

COOKING INSTRUCTIONS:

1. Lay out the whole wheat tortillas on a work surface.

2. Spread 1/2 tablespoon of hummus onto each tortilla.

3. Add 2 ounces of sliced turkey breast onto each tortilla.

4. Top with slices of avocado, bell pepper and red onion.

5. Sprinkle salt and pepper on top of the veggies.

6. Roll up each tortilla tightly.

7. Wrap the tortillas in plastic wrap and store in the fridge.

Cook Time: 15 minutes

Nutritional Value:

This recipe makes four servings. Each serving contains approximately:

Calories: 370 calories; Protein: 25g; Fat: 17g; Carbohydrates: 30g; Fiber: 10g; Sugar: 5g.

Turkey and Avocado Wrap is a healthy and tasty lunch option that can be made in advance and stored in the fridge for easy meal prep. The sliced turkey breast provides a good source of protein, while the avocado adds healthy fats and fiber. The colorful veggies also provide a variety of vitamins and minerals.

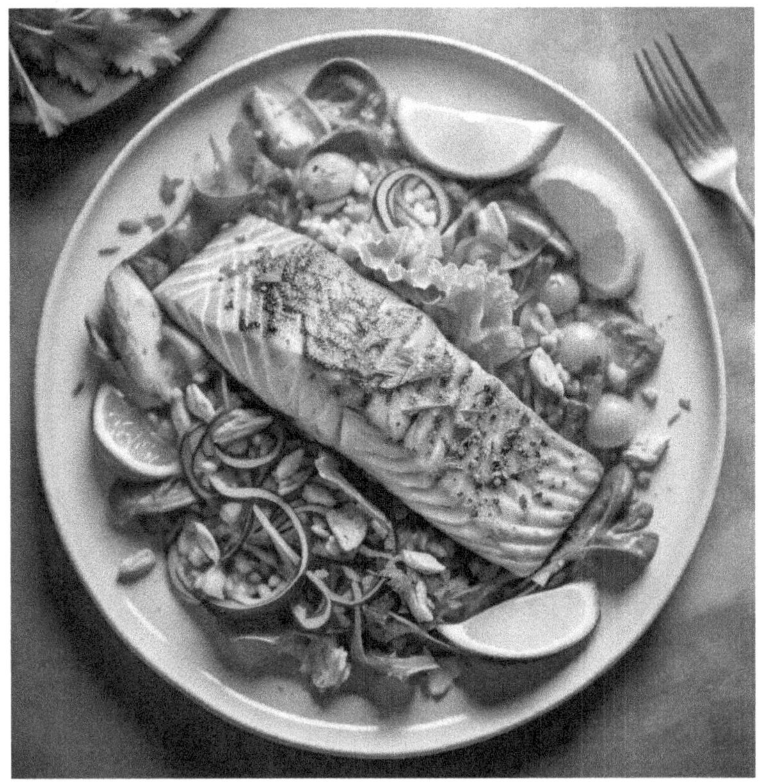

Looking for a flavorful and healthy meal to enjoy during the week? Try this Grilled Salmon Salad! Made with juicy grilled salmon, fresh greens, and a tangy vinaigrette, it's the perfect mix of protein, healthy fats, and vitamins. Plus, it's easy to make and perfect for meal prep!

INGREDIENTS:

- 1 lb salmon fillet

- 6 cups mixed greens (such as spinach, arugula, and lettuce)

- 1/2 cup cherry tomatoes, halved

- 1/4 cup red onion, thinly sliced

- 1/4 cup crumbled feta cheese

- 1/4 cup chopped walnuts

- 1/4 cup olive oil

- 2 tbsp red wine vinegar

- 1 tbsp Dijon mustard

- 1 clove garlic, minced

- Salt and pepper to taste

COOKING INSTRUCTIONS:

1. Season the salmon fillet with salt and pepper.

2. Preheat the grill (or grill pan) to medium-high heat.

3. Grease the grill grates with cooking spray or oil.

4. Place the salmon fillet on the grill, skin side down, and cook for 5-6 minutes per side, or until cooked through.

5. Remove the salmon from the grill and set aside to cool.

6. In a small bowl, whisk together the olive oil, red wine vinegar, Dijon mustard, garlic, salt, and pepper until well combined.

7. In a large mixing bowl, combine the mixed greens, cherry tomatoes, red onion, feta cheese, and chopped walnuts.

8. Add the vinaigrette to the bowl and toss well to coat.

9. Divide the salad into individual meal prep containers.

10. Cut the salmon fillet into portions and add 1 portion to each container.

11. Seal the containers and store in the fridge for up to 4 days.

Prep Time: 20 minutes

Cook Time: 10-12 minutes

NUTRITIONAL VALUE **(per serving):**

Calories: 300; Fat: 25g; Carbohydrates: 6g; Fiber: 2g; Sugar: 2g; Protein: 14g.

This Grilled Salmon Salad Meal Prep is a delicious and healthy option for lunch or dinner. The juicy salmon fillet pairs perfectly with the fresh greens, cherry tomatoes, red onion, and tangy vinaigrette, and it's packed with protein, healthy fats, and vitamins. Give this recipe a try and enjoy the tasty and nutritious benefits of this Grilled Salmon Salad!

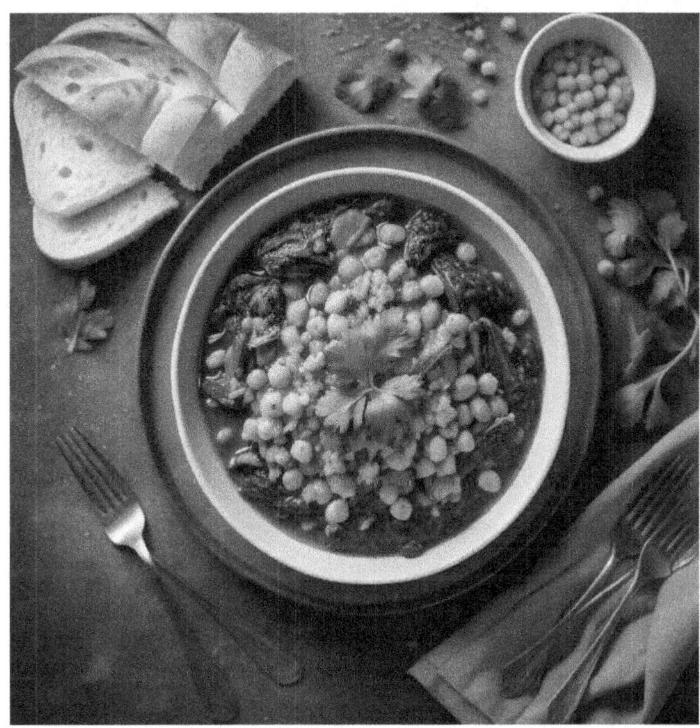

If you're looking for a delicious and nutritious meal that's both satisfying and easy to make, try this Spinach and Chickpea Stew Meal Prep! This hearty and flavorful stew is packed with protein, fiber, and essential nutrients. It's perfect for meal prep and can be enjoyed for lunch or dinner.

INGREDIENTS:

- 1 tbsp olive oil

- 1 large onion, chopped

- 4 cloves of garlic, minced

- 2 cans of chickpeas, drained and rinsed

- 1 can of diced tomatoes

- 1 tbsp tomato paste

- 1 tsp smoked paprika

- 1 tsp ground cumin

- 1 tsp ground coriander

- 1/2 tsp chili powder

- 4 cups vegetable broth

- 1/2 cup quinoa

- 4 cups fresh spinach

- Salt and pepper to taste

COOKING INSTRUCTIONS:

1. Heat the olive oil in a large pot over medium heat.

2. Add the chopped onions and minced garlic, and cook until softened, about 5 minutes.

3. Add the chickpeas, diced tomatoes, tomato paste, smoked paprika, cumin, coriander, and chili powder. Stir well to combine.

4. Add the vegetable broth and quinoa. Bring the mixture to a boil, then reduce the heat and simmer for 20-25 minutes, or until the quinoa is cooked and the stew has thickened.

5. Add the spinach to the pot and stir until wilted, about 2-3 minutes.

6. Season with salt and pepper to taste.

7. Divide the stew into individual meal prep containers.

8. Allow the containers to cool to room temperature before sealing them and storing them in the fridge for up to 4 days.

Prep Time: 10 minutes

Cook Time: 30 minutes

NUTRITIONAL VALUE **(per serving):**

Calories: 346; Fat: 7g; Carbohydrates: 55g; Fiber: 14g; Sugar: 10g; Protein: 16g.

This Spinach and Chickpea Stew Meal Prep is a healthy and delicious way to stay full and satisfied throughout the day. The chickpeas provide a good source of plant-based protein and fiber, while the spinach adds essential nutrients to the mix. Plus, this recipe is easy to make and perfect for meal prep, making it a great option for busy weeks. Give it a try and enjoy this flavorful and nutritious stew!

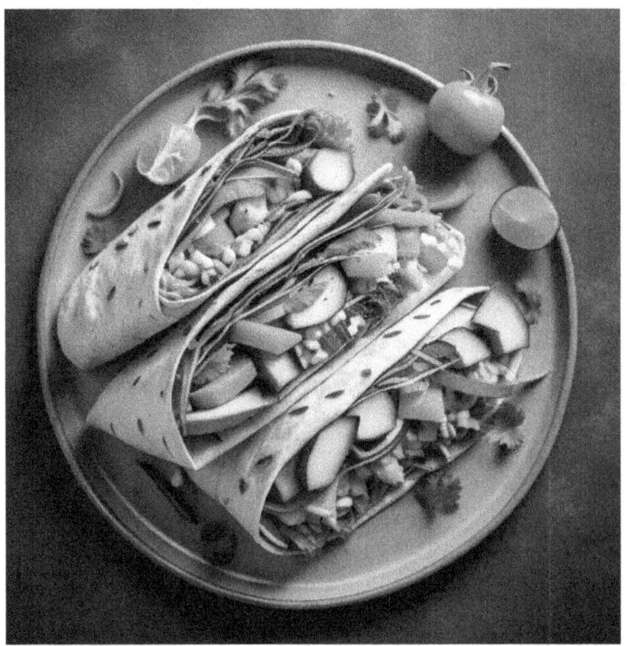

Need a quick and easy meal option for the week? Try this Veggie Wrap! Filled with fresh vegetables, hummus, and avocado, it's a delicious and healthy alternative to traditional sandwich options. Plus, it's easy to make and perfect for meal prep!

INGREDIENTS:

- 5 whole wheat wraps

- 1 cucumber, sliced

- 1 bell pepper, sliced

- 1 carrot, grated

- 1 avocado, sliced

- 1/2 cup hummus

- 1/4 cup chopped fresh herbs (such as parsley or cilantro)

- Salt and pepper to taste

1. Lay out the whole wheat wraps on a clean work surface.

2. Spread each wrap with 1-2 tablespoons of hummus, leaving a 1-inch border around the edges.

3. Divide the sliced cucumber, bell pepper, and grated carrot between the 5 wraps, arranging the vegetables in a line down the center of each wrap.

4. Add the sliced avocado and chopped herbs to each wrap.

5. Season each wrap with salt and pepper to taste.

6. Roll each wrap tightly, folding in the edges as you go, until you have a neat and compact roll.

7. Cut each wrap in half or into bite-sized pieces.

8. Divide the wraps into individual meal prep containers.

9. Seal the containers and store in the fridge for up to 4 days.

Prep Time: 10 minutes

Cook Time: N/A

NUTRITIONAL VALUE **(per serving):**

Calories: 300; Fat: 15g; Carbohydrates: 34g; Fiber: 11g; Sugar: 6g; Protein: 10g.

This Veggie Wrap Meal Prep is a delicious and healthy option for lunch or dinner. The fresh vegetables and creamy hummus and avocado provide a satisfying balance of nutrients, and it's a perfect alternative to traditional sandwich options. Give this recipe a try and enjoy the tasty and nutritious benefits of this flavorful Veggie Wrap!

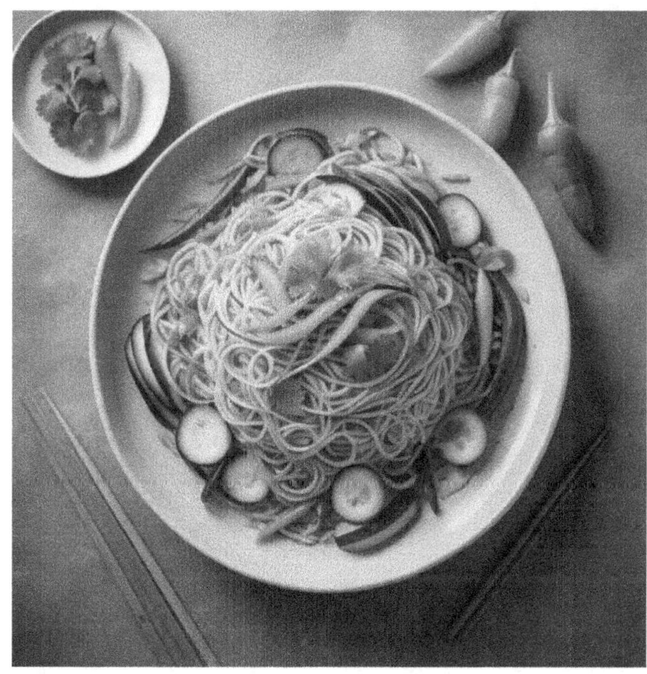

Looking for a tasty and refreshing meal for the week? Try this Soba Noodle Salad! Made with fresh vegetables and tender soba noodles, this salad is bursting with flavor and nutrition. Plus, it's easy to make and perfect for meal prep!

INGREDIENTS:

- 8 oz soba noodles

- 1 cucumber, julienned

- 1 bell pepper, julienned

- 1 carrot, julienned

- 1/4 cup chopped scallions

- 1/2 cup chopped fresh herbs (such as cilantro and mint)

- 1/4 cup toasted sesame seeds

- 1/2 cup rice vinegar

- 2 tbsp soy sauce or tamari

- 2 tbsp honey or maple syrup

- 1 clove garlic, minced

- Salt and pepper to taste

COOKING INSTRUCTIONS:

1. Cook the soba noodles according to package instructions, then rinse under cold water and drain well.

2. In a large bowl, combine the julienned cucumber, bell pepper, and carrot, along with the chopped scallions, fresh herbs, and toasted sesame seeds.

3. In a separate bowl, whisk together the rice vinegar, soy sauce or tamari, honey or maple syrup, minced garlic, salt, and pepper to make the dressing.

4. Add the cooked and cooled soba noodles to the vegetable mixture, then pour in the dressing and toss well to combine.

5. Divide the salad into individual meal prep containers.

6. Allow the salad to cool to room temperature before sealing the containers and storing them in the fridge for up to 4 days.

7. To serve, simply give the salad a quick toss and enjoy!

Prep Time: 15 minutes

Cook Time: 10 minutes

 (per serving):

Calories: 300; Fat: 7g; Carbohydrates: 53g; Fiber: 5g; Sugar: 11g; Protein: 1g.

This Soba Noodle Salad Meal Prep is a perfect option for a light and refreshing lunch or dinner. The fresh vegetables and tender soba noodles offer a fantastic balance of nutrition and flavor, and the dressing adds a delightful zing of sweet and salty flavor. Give this recipe a try and enjoy the delicious and nutritious benefits of this delightful Soba Noodle Salad!

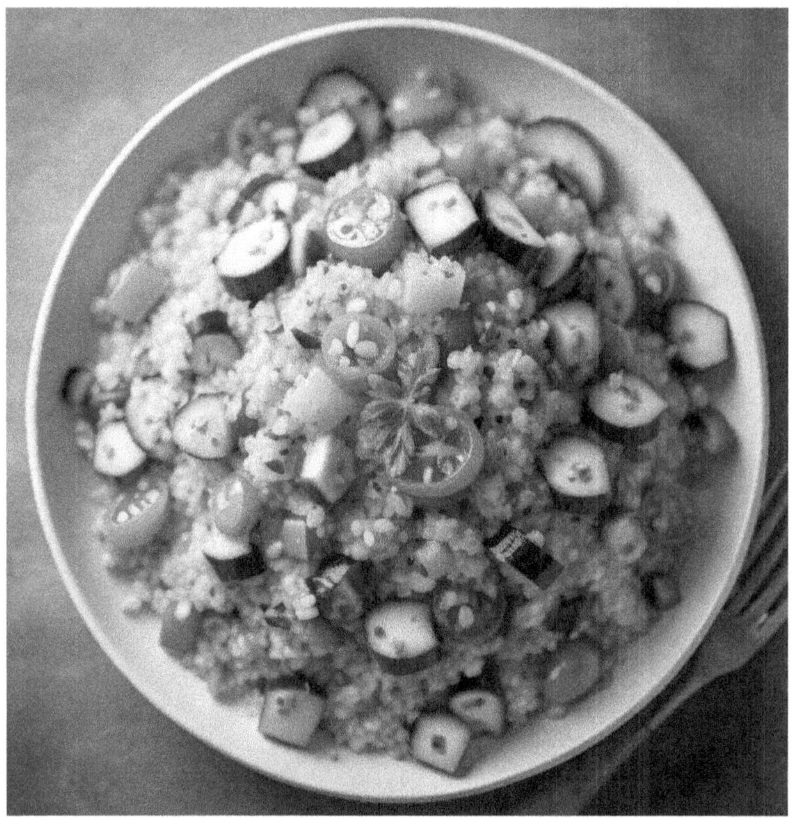

Looking for a satisfying and nutritious meal for the week? Try this Quinoa Salad! Loaded with fresh vegetables and protein-packed quinoa, this salad is a delicious and healthy option for lunch or dinner. Plus, it's simple to make and perfect for meal prep!

INGREDIENTS:

- 1 cup quinoa, rinsed

- 2 cups water or vegetable broth

- 1 red bell pepper, diced

- 1 yellow bell pepper, diced

- 1 cucumber, diced

- 1/2 red onion, diced

- 1 cup cherry tomatoes, halved

- 1/4 cup chopped fresh herbs (such as parsley or cilantro)

- 1/4 cup olive oil

- 2 tbsp red wine vinegar

- 1 tbsp Dijon mustard

- Salt and pepper to taste

COOKING INSTRUCTIONS:

1. In a medium saucepan, combine the quinoa and water or vegetable broth. Bring to a boil, then reduce heat to a simmer and cover. Cook for 15-20 minutes, or until the liquid is absorbed and the quinoa is tender.

2. While the quinoa is cooking, prepare the vegetables and herbs, and make the dressing.

3. In a large bowl, combine the cooked quinoa, diced bell peppers, cucumber, red onion, cherry tomatoes, and chopped herbs.

4. In a separate bowl, whisk together the olive oil, red wine vinegar, Dijon mustard, salt, and pepper to make the dressing.

5. Pour the dressing over the quinoa and vegetable mixture, and toss well to combine.

6. Divide the salad into individual meal prep containers.

7. Allow the salad to cool to room temperature before sealing the containers and storing them in the fridge for up to 4 days.

8. To serve, simply give the salad a quick toss and enjoy!

Prep Time: 10 minutes

Cook Time: 20 minutes

NUTRITIONAL VALUE **(per serving):**

Calories: 320; Fat: 14g; Carbohydrates: 39g; Fiber: 6g; Sugar: 5g; Protein: 8g.

This Quinoa Salad Meal Prep is a tasty and healthy option for lunch or dinner. The protein-packed quinoa and fresh vegetables provide a nutritious and satisfying meal, and the dressing adds a delightful tangy flavor. Give this recipe a try and enjoy the delicious and nutritious benefits of this fantastic Quinoa Salad!

DINNERS

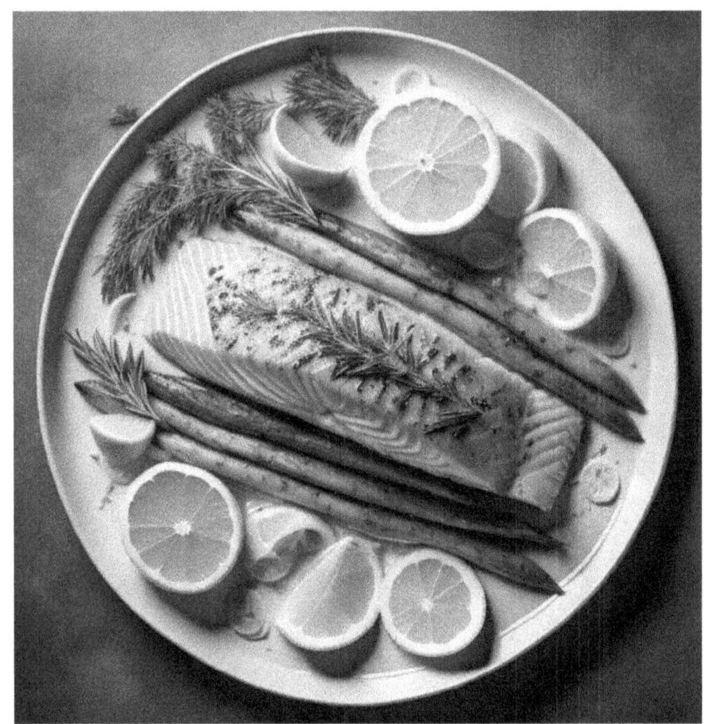

Baked Salmon with Lemon and Herbs is a delicious and healthy meal prep that is perfect for dinner. This dish is rich in omega-3 fatty acids, protein, and micronutrients, making it a nutritious and satisfying option.

INGREDIENTS:

- 4 salmon fillets

- 2 tablespoons olive oil

- 1 lemon, sliced

- 1 tablespoon chopped fresh herbs (such as thyme or parsley)

- Salt and pepper, to taste

1. Preheat the oven to 400°F.

2. Line a baking dish with parchment paper.

3. Brush olive oil onto the salmon fillets.

4. Place the salmon fillets in the baking dish.

5. Season the salmon fillets with salt, pepper, and chopped herbs.

6. Top each salmon fillet with a lemon slice.

7. Bake for 12-15 minutes, or until the salmon is cooked through.

8. Let the salmon cool for a few minutes before packing into meal prep containers.

Cook Time: 20 minutes

Nutritional Value:

This recipe makes four servings. Each serving contains approximately:

Calories: 350 calories; Protein: 35g; Fat: 20g; Carbohydrates: 5g; Fiber: 1g; Sugar: 1g.

Baked Salmon with Lemon and Herbs is a healthy and delicious meal prep option that can be made in advance and reheated for easy dinners. The salmon provides a good source of omega-3 fatty acids, while the herbs and lemon add flavor and micronutrients. Serve the salmon with a side of roasted veggies or quinoa for a complete meal.

8. LENTIL SHEPHERD'S PIE WITH SWEET POTATO TOPPING

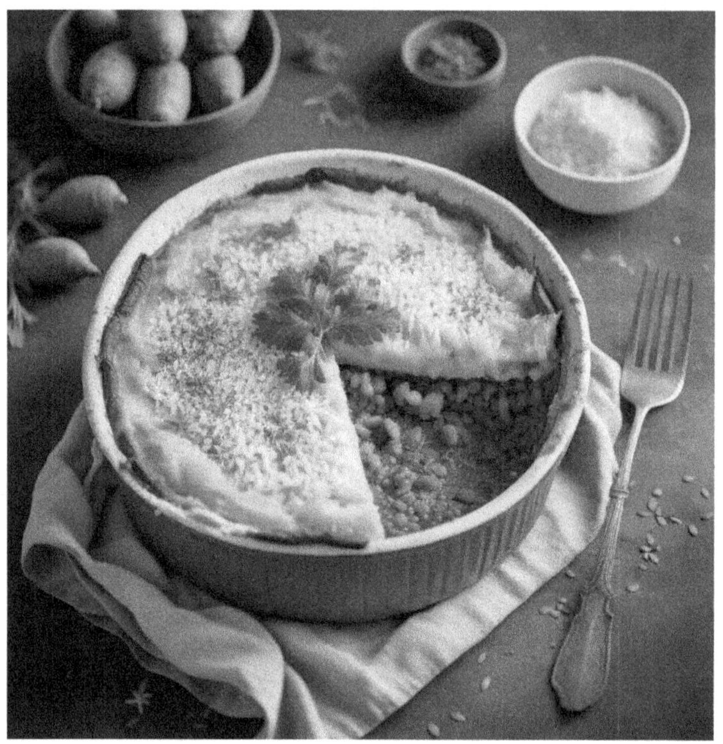

Lentil Shepherd's Pie with Sweet Potato Topping is a hearty and flavorful meal prep that is perfect for a cold winter evening. This twist on a classic dish is packed with plant-based protein, fiber, and nutrients, making it a healthy and satisfying option.

INGREDIENTS:

- 2 cups green or brown lentils, cooked

- 2 large sweet potatoes, peeled and diced

- 1 onion, chopped

- 2 garlic cloves, minced

- 2 carrots, peeled and chopped

- 2 celery stalks, chopped

- 1 tablespoon olive oil

- 2 tablespoons tomato paste

- 2 cups vegetable broth

- 1 teaspoon dried thyme

- Salt and pepper, to taste

COOKING INSTRUCTIONS:

1. Preheat the oven to 375°F.

2. In a large skillet, heat the olive oil over medium heat.

3. Add the onion and garlic and cook until softened.

4. Add the carrots and celery and cook for another 5 minutes.

5. Add the cooked lentils, tomato paste, vegetable broth, thyme, salt, and pepper to the skillet. Stir to combine.

6. Bring the mixture to a boil, then reduce the heat and simmer for 10 minutes.

7. While the lentil mixture is simmering, cook the sweet potato in a separate pot until tender.

8. Mash the cooked sweet potato and season with salt and pepper.

9. Transfer the lentil mixture to a baking dish and spread the mashed sweet potato on top.

10. Bake for 25-30 minutes, or until the sweet potato is lightly browned on top.

11. Allow the lentil shepherd's pie to cool before dividing it into meal prep containers.

Cook Time: 1 hour

NUTRITIONAL VALUE:

This recipe makes four servings. Each serving contains approximately:

Calories: 450 calories; Protein: 20g; Fat: 8g; Carbohydrates: 80g; Fiber: 20g; Sugar: 18g.

Lentil Shepherd's Pie with Sweet Potato Topping is a flavorful and nutritious meal prep that is perfect for a comforting winter dinner. The lentils provide a good source of plant-based protein and fiber, while the sweet potato topping adds micronutrients and natural sweetness. Serve the shepherd's pie with a green salad or steamed veggies for a complete meal.

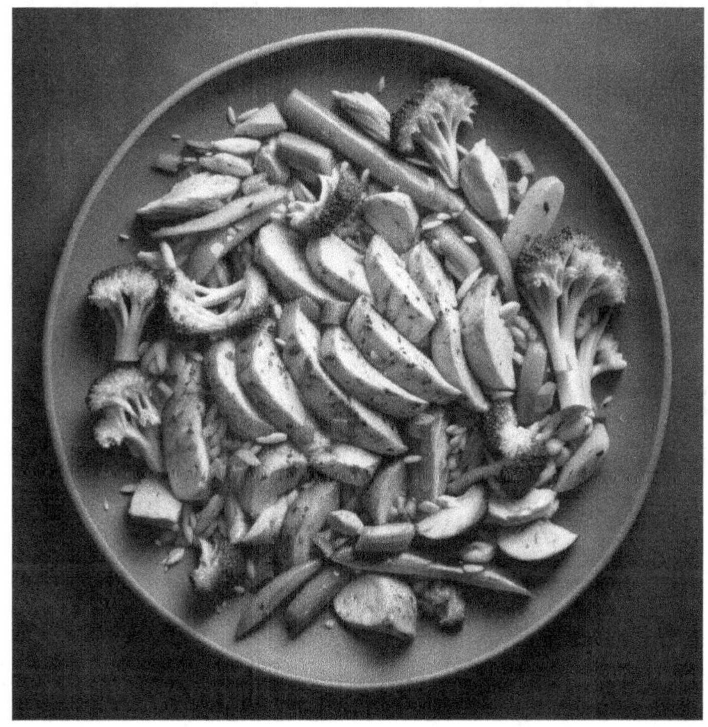

Chicken and Vegetable Stir-Fry is a delicious and healthy meal prep option that is perfect for a busy week. This dish is packed with lean protein, veggies, and flavors, making it a nutritious and satisfying option.

INGREDIENTS:

- 2 chicken breasts, sliced

- 2 tablespoons olive oil

- 1 onion, sliced

- 2 garlic cloves, minced

- 2 carrots, peeled and sliced

- 1 red bell pepper, sliced

- 1 green bell pepper, sliced

- 1 cup snow peas

- 1 tablespoon cornstarch

- 1/4 cup soy sauce

- 1/4 cup honey

- 2 tablespoons rice vinegar

- Salt and pepper, to taste

COOKING INSTRUCTIONS:

1. In a large skillet or wok, heat the olive oil over medium-high heat.

2. Add the chicken and cook until browned on all sides. Remove the chicken from the skillet and set it aside.

3. In the same skillet, add the onion and garlic and cook until softened.

4. Add the carrots, bell peppers, and snow peas to the skillet and cook until tender-crisp.

5. Combine the cornstarch, soy sauce, honey, and rice vinegar in a bowl. Stir to combine.

6. Add the cooked chicken back to the skillet and pour the sauce over everything. Stir to combine.

7. Cook for another 2-3 minutes, or until the sauce has thickened and everything is heated through.

8. Allow the stir-fry to cool before dividing it into meal prep containers.

Cook Time: 30 minutes

NUTRITIONAL VALUE:

This recipe makes four servings. Each serving contains approximately:

Calories: 400 calories; Protein: 30g; Fat: 12g; Carbohydrates: 45g; Fiber: 5g; Sugar: 25g.

Chicken and Vegetable Stir-Fry is a delicious and colorful meal prep that can be made in advance and reheated for easy dinners. The chicken provides a good source of lean protein, while the veggies add fiber and micronutrients. Serve the stir-fry with brown rice or quinoa for a complete meal.

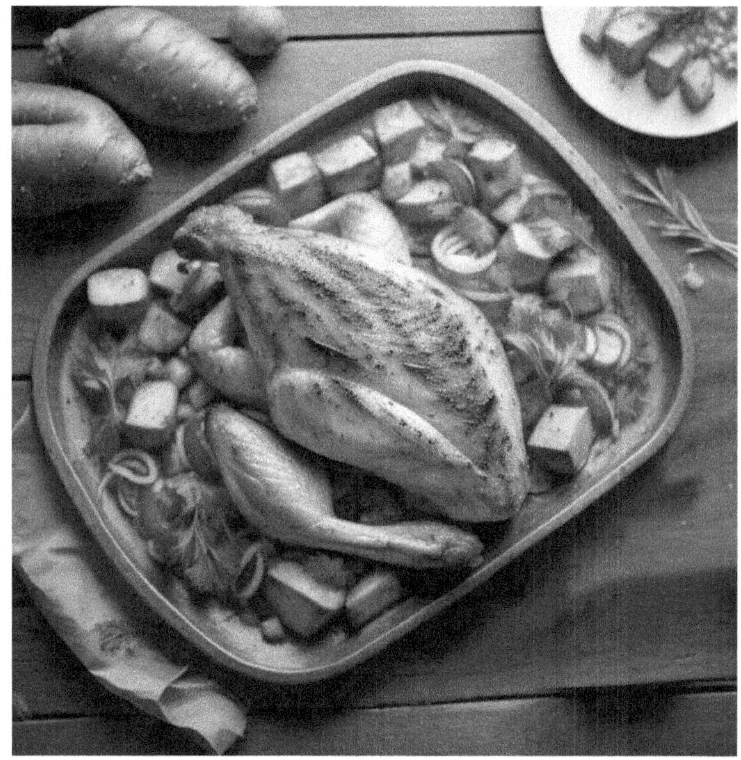

Looking for a delicious and easy-to-prepare meal for the week ahead? Try this Baked Chicken and Sweet Potato recipe! This meal is packed with protein and healthy carbs, making it a great option for a post-workout meal. Plus, it's easy to make and perfect for meal prep!

INGREDIENTS:

- 4 boneless, skinless chicken breasts

- 4 medium sweet potatoes, peeled and cubed

- 1 tbsp olive oil

- 1 tsp garlic powder

- 1 tsp paprika

- Salt and pepper to taste

1. Preheat the oven to 400°F (200°C).

2. In a large bowl, toss the cubed sweet potatoes with the olive oil, garlic powder, paprika, salt, and pepper until well coated.

3. Arrange the sweet potatoes in a single layer on a large baking sheet.

4. Place the chicken breasts on top of the sweet potatoes.

5. Season the chicken breasts with additional salt, pepper, and paprika, as desired.

6. Bake for 25-30 minutes, or until the chicken is cooked through and the sweet potatoes are tender and golden brown.

7. Let the chicken and sweet potatoes cool for a few minutes, then divide them into individual meal prep containers.

8. Allow the containers to cool to room temperature before sealing them and storing them in the fridge for up to 4 days.

9. To serve, simply reheat the containers in the microwave or oven.

Prep Time: 10 minutes

Cook Time: 25-30 minutes

NUTRITIONAL VALUE (per serving):

Calories: 380; Fat: 7g; Carbohydrates: 44g; Fiber: 6g; Sugar: 9g; Protein: 37g.

This Baked Chicken and Sweet Potato Meal Prep is an easy and delicious option for a healthy and satisfying meal. The chicken is tender and flavorful, and the sweet potatoes are perfectly seasoned and soft. This recipe is also high in protein and healthy carbs, making it a great option for post-workout meals or anytime you need a nutritious and filling meal. Give it a try and enjoy the delicious and healthy benefits of this fantastic dish!

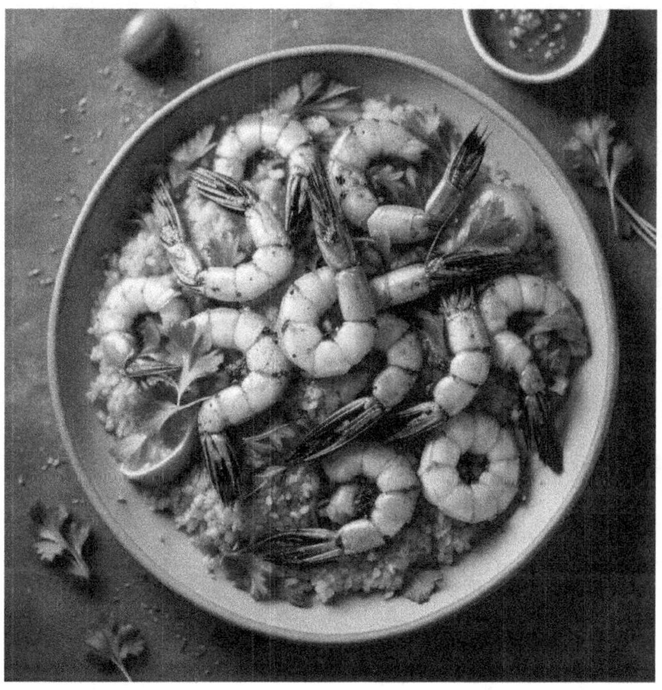

Looking for a light and healthy meal for the week ahead? Try this Grilled Shrimp and Quinoa recipe! Packed with protein and fresh flavors, this meal is perfect for lunch or dinner. Plus, it's easy to make and perfect for meal prep!

INGREDIENTS:

- 1 lb large shrimp, peeled and deveined

- 1 cup quinoa, rinsed

- 2 cups water or vegetable broth

- 1 red bell pepper, diced

- 1 yellow bell pepper, diced

- 1/2 red onion, diced

- 1/4 cup chopped fresh herbs (such as parsley or cilantro)

- 1/4 cup olive oil

- 2 tbsp red wine vinegar

- Salt and pepper to taste

COOKING INSTRUCTIONS:

1. In a medium saucepan, combine the quinoa and water or vegetable broth. Bring to a boil, then reduce heat to a simmer and cover. Cook for 15-20 minutes, or until the liquid is absorbed and the quinoa is tender.

2. While the quinoa is cooking, prepare the vegetables, herbs, and shrimp, and heat up your grill or grill pan.

3. In a large bowl, combine the diced bell peppers, red onion, chopped herbs, olive oil, red wine vinegar, salt, and pepper. Mix well to make the marinade.

4. Add the shrimp to the marinade, and toss well to coat.

5. Thread the shrimp onto skewers, or place them on a grill pan.

6. Grill the shrimp over medium-high heat for 3-4 minutes per side, or until cooked through and slightly charred.

7. Once the quinoa is cooked, fluff it with a fork and add it to the bowl with the vegetables. Mix well to combine.

8. Divide the shrimp and quinoa mixture into individual meal prep containers.

9. Allow the containers to cool to room temperature before sealing them and storing them in the fridge for up to 4 days.

10. To serve, simply reheat the containers in the microwave or eat the meal cold.

Prep Time: 20 minutes

Cook Time: 20-25 minutes

NUTRITIONAL VALUE **(per serving):**

Calories: 330; Fat: 15g; Carbohydrates: 21g; Fiber: 4g; Sugar: 4g; Protein: 25g.

This Grilled Shrimp and Quinoa Meal Prep is a light and healthy option for lunch or dinner that's packed with fresh flavors and protein. The shrimp is juicy and flavorful, and the quinoa is fluffy and filling. Plus, this recipe is easy to make and perfect for meal prep, so you can enjoy a delicious and nutritious meal all week long. Give it a try and enjoy the tasty and healthy benefits!

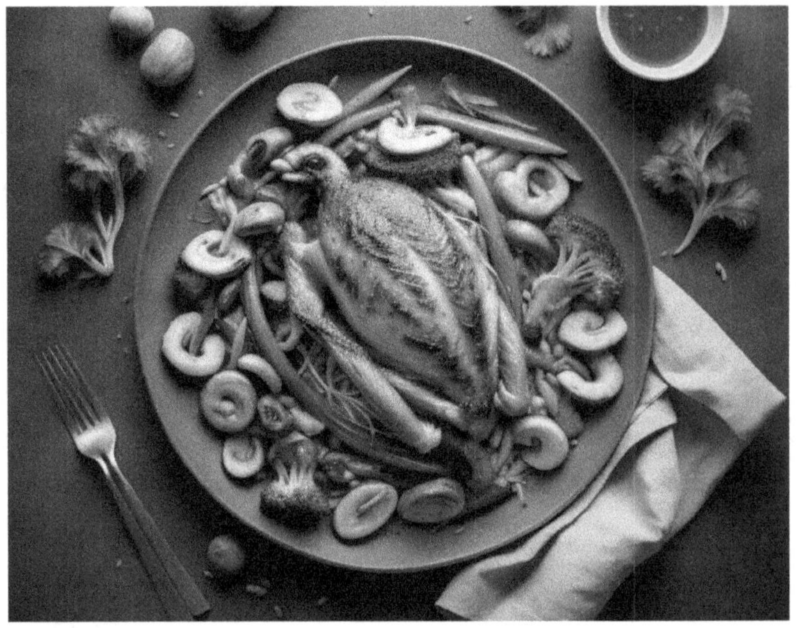

Looking for a healthy and delicious meal for the week ahead? Try this Turkey and Mushroom Stir-Fry recipe! This meal is high in protein and full of veggies, making it a great option for lunch or dinner. Plus, it's easy to make and perfect for meal prep!

INGREDIENTS:

- 1 lb ground turkey

- 1 lb mushrooms, sliced

- 1 red bell pepper, sliced

- 1 yellow onion, sliced

- 3 cloves garlic, minced

- 2 tbsp soy sauce

- 2 tbsp olive oil

- Salt and pepper to taste

1. Heat the olive oil in a large skillet over medium-high heat.

2. Add the ground turkey and cook, breaking it up with a wooden spoon, until browned and cooked through, about 7-8 minutes.

3. Remove the turkey from the skillet and set it aside.

4. Add the sliced mushrooms to the skillet and sauté for 5-6 minutes, until they are soft and browned.

5. Add the sliced bell pepper, onion, and minced garlic to the skillet with the mushrooms. Stir well to combine.

6. Cook the vegetables for 5-6 minutes, or until they are tender and slightly charred.

7. Add the cooked ground turkey back to the skillet, and stir well to combine.

8. Add the soy sauce, salt, and pepper to taste, and mix well.

9. Divide the stir-fry into individual meal prep containers.

10. Allow the containers to cool to room temperature before sealing them and storing them in the fridge for up to 4 days.

11. To serve, simply reheat the containers in the microwave or in a skillet on the stove.

Prep Time: 15 minutes

Cook Time: 25 minutes

 (per serving):

Calories: 300; Fat: 14g; Carbohydrates: 9g; Fiber: 2g; Sugar: 4g; Protein: 34g

This Turkey and Mushroom Stir-Fry Meal Prep is a healthy and flavorful option for lunch or dinner that's packed with protein and veggies. The turkey is juicy and tender, and the mushrooms, bell pepper, and onion add a delicious crunch and flavor. Plus, this recipe is easy to make and perfect for meal prep, so you can have a nutritious and satisfying meal ready in no time. Give it a try and enjoy the tasty and healthy benefits!

6. SPAGHETTI SQUASH WITH VEGGIE MEATBALLS

If you're looking for a comforting and healthy meal that's not only delicious but also low in carbs, try this Spaghetti Squash with Veggie Meatballs recipe. This meal is sure to satisfy your cravings without making you feel guilty. It's also perfect for meal prep and can be easily customized to fit your preferences.

INGREDIENTS:

- 1 medium spaghetti squash, halved and seeded

- 1 cup of your favorite marinara sauce

- 1 package of frozen veggie meatballs

- 1 cup chopped spinach

- 1/2 cup chopped red onion

- 2 cloves minced garlic

- 2 tbsp olive oil

- Salt and pepper to taste

- Grated Parmesan cheese for topping (optional)

COOKING INSTRUCTIONS:

1. Preheat the oven to 375°F (190°C).

2. Brush the cut sides of the spaghetti squash with olive oil. Place on a baking sheet cut-side down and roast for 30-40 minutes or until tender.

3. While the squash is roasting, prepare the veggie meatballs according to package instructions, set aside.

4. Heat olive oil in a pan over medium heat, add red onion and sauté for 3-5 minutes. Add minced garlic and cook for an additional 30 seconds.

5. Add the spinach to the pan and cook until wilted, about 3 minutes.

6. Add the marinara sauce and cooked veggie meatballs to the pan. Stir to combine and let it simmer for 5 minutes.

7. Once the spaghetti squash is cooked, use a fork to scrape the flesh from the sides to create "spaghetti" strands.

8. Top each spaghetti squash half with the marinara veggie meatballs mixture.

9. If desired, sprinkle with grated Parmesan cheese.

10. Divide into individual meal prep containers.

11. Allow the containers to cool to room temperature before sealing them and storing them in the fridge for up to 4 days.

12. To serve, simply reheat the containers in the microwave or in a skillet on the stove.

Prep Time: 10 minutes

Cook Time: 45 minutes

NUTRITIONAL VALUE **(per serving):**

Calories: 330; Fat: 19g; Carbohydrates: 27g; Fiber: 7g; Sugar: 12g; Protein: 13g

This Spaghetti Squash with Veggie Meatballs Meal Prep is a healthy and flavorful option for lunch or dinner that's low in carbs and high in nutrients. The spaghetti squash provides a good source of fiber, while the veggie meatballs offer a protein-rich base. Plus, this recipe is easy to make and perfect for meal prep, making it a great option for busy weeks. Give it a try and enjoy the tasty and healthy benefits!

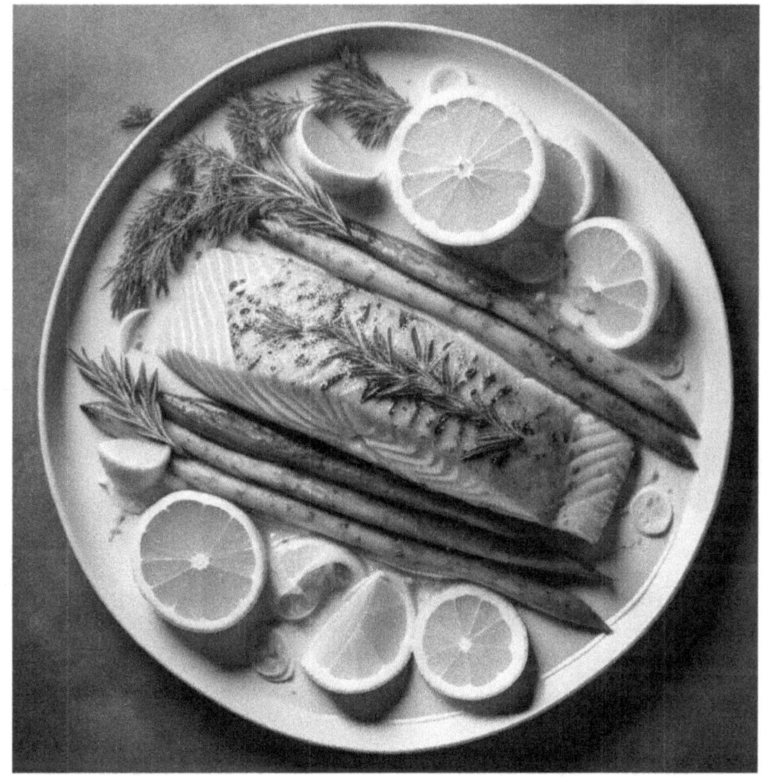

Looking for a meal that's both delicious and nutritious? Try this Baked Salmon and Asparagus Meal Prep! This dish is packed with nutrients, high in protein, and incredibly flavorful. It's perfect for meal prep and guaranteed to satisfy your appetite.

INGREDIENTS:

- 4 (6oz) salmon fillets

- 1 lb of asparagus, trimmed

- 1 lemon, sliced

- 2 tbsp olive oil

- Salt and pepper to taste

- Fresh thyme for garnish (optional)

1. Preheat the oven to 375°F (190°C).

2. Place the salmon fillets on a baking sheet lined with parchment paper.

3. Arrange the asparagus around the salmon on the baking sheet.

4. Drizzle olive oil over the salmon and asparagus. Season with salt and pepper.

5. Place the slices of lemon over the salmon fillets.

6. Bake for 12-15 minutes, or until the salmon is cooked through and the asparagus is tender.

7. Divide the salmon and asparagus into individual meal prep containers.

8. Allow the containers to cool to room temperature before sealing them and storing them in the fridge for up to 4 days.

9. Garnish with fresh thyme (optional).

Prep Time: 10 minutes

Cook Time: 15 minutes

NUTRITIONAL VALUE **(per serving):**

Calories: 408; Fat: 26g; Carbohydrates: 6g; Fiber: 3g; Sugar: 2g; Protein: 39g.

This Baked Salmon and Asparagus Meal Prep is a healthy and satisfying meal that's perfect for lunch or dinner. The salmon fillets are packed with healthy omega-3 fats and high-quality protein, while the asparagus provides a good source of fiber and other essential nutrients. Plus, this recipe is easy to make and perfect for meal prep, making it a great option for busy weeks. Give it a try and enjoy the tasty and healthy benefits!

CHAPTER 6

DESSERTS

1. BANANA BREAD WITH WALNUTS AND CHIA SEEDS

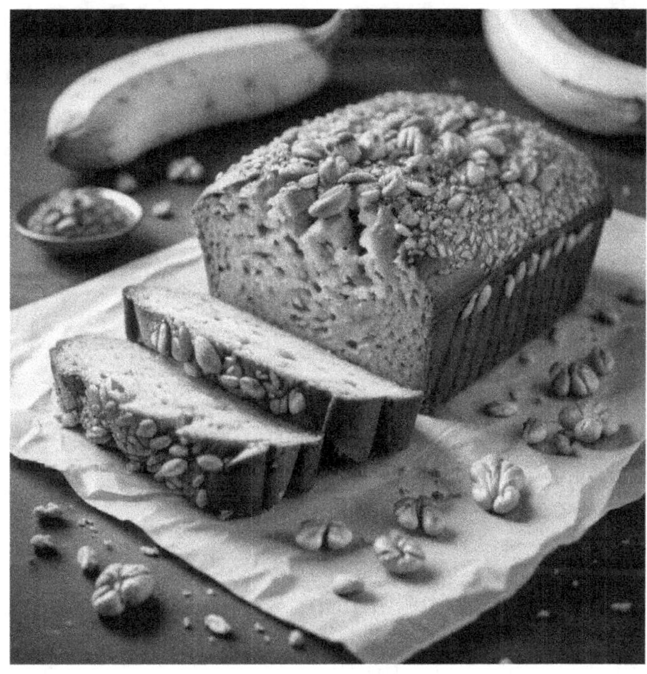

Banana Bread with Walnuts and Chia Seeds is a delicious dessert that is perfect for a sweet treat or quick breakfast. This recipe is packed with fiber, healthy fats, and natural sweetness, making it a healthier alternative to traditional banana bread.

INGREDIENTS:

- 4 ripe bananas, mashed

- 2 eggs, beaten

- 2 cups almond flour

- 1/4 cup chia seeds

- 1/4 cup chopped walnuts

- 1/4 cup honey

- 1/4 cup coconut oil, melted

- 1 teaspoon baking soda

- 1 teaspoon cinnamon

- 1/2 teaspoon salt

1. Preheat the oven to 350°F.

2. In a large bowl, combine the mashed bananas, eggs, honey, and coconut oil. Stir to combine.

3. In a separate bowl, combine the almond flour, chia seeds, chopped walnuts, baking soda, cinnamon, and salt. Stir to combine.

4. Add the dry ingredients to the wet ingredients and stir until everything is mixed together.

5. Grease a loaf pan with coconut oil and pour the batter into the pan.

6. Bake for 50-60 minutes, or until a toothpick inserted in the center comes out clean.

7. Let the banana bread cool before slicing it and dividing it into meal prep containers.

Cook Time: 1 hour

This recipe makes eight servings. Each serving contains approximately:

Calories: 310 calories; Protein: 8g; Fat: 22g; Carbohydrates: 22g; Fiber: 6g; Sugar: 11g.

Banana Bread with Walnuts and Chia Seeds is a delicious and nutritious dessert that is perfect for meal prep. The almond flour and chia seeds add fiber and healthy fats, while the bananas and honey provide natural sweetness. Serve the banana bread with a dollop of plain Greek yogurt or almond butter for an extra dose of protein and healthy fats.

2. CHOCOLATE AVOCADO MOUSSE

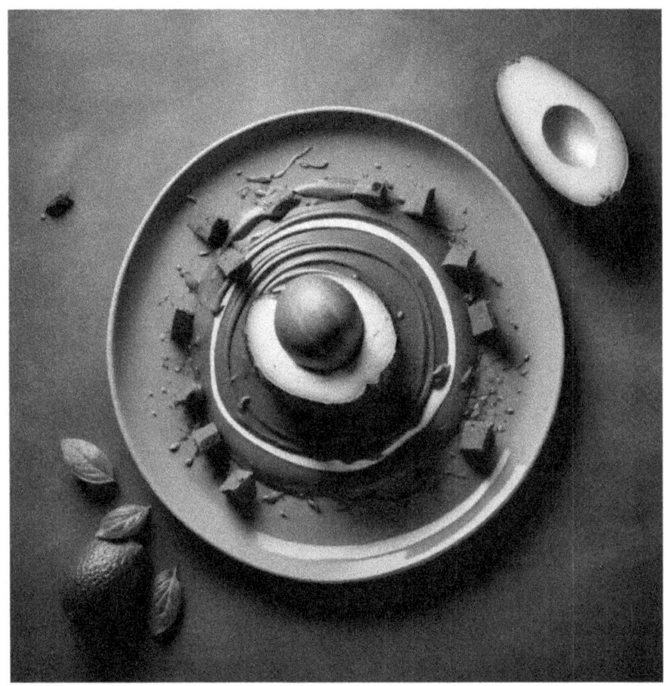

Chocolate Avocado Mousse is a decadent and creamy dessert that is perfect for satisfying your sweet tooth or impressing dinner guests. This recipe is made with healthy ingredients, including ripe avocados and dark chocolate, making it an indulgent yet nutritious treat.

INGREDIENTS:

- 2 ripe avocados, pitted and peeled

- 1/2 cup dark chocolate chips

- 1/2 cup unsweetened almond milk

- 1/4 cup raw honey or maple syrup

- 1 teaspoon vanilla extract

- Pinch of sea salt

- Optional toppings: fresh fruit, coconut whipped cream, chopped nuts, or cocoa powder.

1. In a small saucepan, melt the dark chocolate chips and almond milk over low heat, stirring occasionally.

2. Once melted, remove from heat and allow to cool to room temperature.

3. In a blender or food processor, combine the cooled chocolate mixture, ripe avocados, honey, vanilla extract, and sea salt. Blend until smooth and creamy, scraping down the sides as needed.

4. Divide the chocolate avocado mousse into individual serving containers, and refrigerate for at least 2 hours or until firm.

5. Before serving, add desired toppings such as fresh fruit, coconut whipped cream, chopped nuts, or cocoa powder.

Cook Time: 10-15 minutes

Nutritional Value:

This recipe makes six servings. Each serving contains approximately:

Calories: 220 calories; Protein: 3g; Fat: 16g; Carbohydrates: 23g; Fiber: 5g; Sugar: 16g.

Chocolate Avocado Mousse is a delicious and satisfying dessert that is perfect for a meal prep. Avocado provides healthy fats, while dark chocolate adds antioxidants and natural sweetness. Serve the mousse with fresh fruit, whipped cream, or chopped nuts for an extra texture and flavor.

3. BERRY CRUMBLE WITH OATMEAL TOPPING

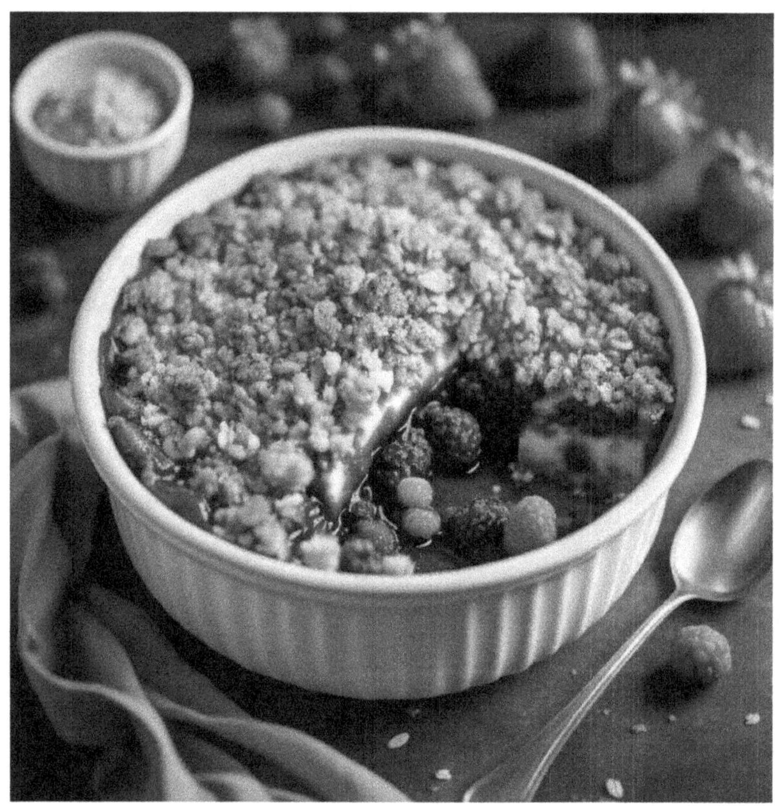

Berry Crumble with Oatmeal Topping is a delicious and healthier dessert that is perfect for a sweet treat or after-dinner indulgence. Made with a mix of fresh berries and a crunchy oatmeal topping, this recipe is packed with fiber, vitamins, and antioxidants.

INGREDIENTS:

- 4 cups mixed berries (raspberries, blueberries, strawberries, blackberries)

- 1/4 cup honey

- 1/4 cup almond flour

- 1/4 cup rolled oats

- 1/4 cup chopped walnuts

- 1/4 cup coconut oil, melted

- 1 teaspoon cinnamon

- Pinch of sea salt

COOKING INSTRUCTIONS:

1. Preheat the oven to 350°F.

2. In a large bowl, mix together the mixed berries and honey.

3. Pour the berry mixture in a baking dish and set aside.

4. In a separate bowl, mix together the almond flour, rolled oats, chopped walnuts, melted coconut oil, cinnamon, and sea salt.

5. Stir the oatmeal mixture well, and evenly sprinkle it over the berry mixture.

6. Bake for 25-30 minutes, or until the berry mixture is bubbling and the crumble is golden brown.

7. Let the berry crumble cool for 10-15 minutes before serving.

8. Divide the crumble into serving containers for meal prep.

Cook Time: 30 minutes

Nutritional Value:

This recipe makes eight servings. Each serving contains approximately:

Calories: 190 calories; Protein: 2g; Fat: 11g; Carbohydrates: 22g; Fiber: 4g; Sugar: 16g.

Berry Crumble with Oatmeal Topping is a delicious and healthier alternative to traditional fruit desserts. The mix of fresh berries provides natural sweetness and antioxidants, while the oatmeal topping adds fiber and crunch. Serve the crumble with a dollop of plain Greek yogurt or whipped cream for an extra flavor.

4. BAKED APPLE RECIPE

Looking for a simple and tasty dessert that's also healthy? Try this Baked Apples recipe! These apples are easy to make and packed with flavor, and they can be enjoyed on their own or with a scoop of vanilla ice cream.

INGREDIENTS:

- 4 medium-sized apples (use a firm variety like Granny Smith or Honeycrisp)

- 2 tbsp butter (or coconut oil for a vegan option)

- 2 tbsp brown sugar (or coconut sugar for a healthier option)

- 1 tsp cinnamon

- 1/4 cup chopped walnuts (optional)

COOKING INSTRUCTIONS:

1. Preheat the oven to 375°F (190°C).

2. Cut off the top of each apple and use a spoon or melon baller to scoop out the core and seeds, leaving the bottom intact.

3. Place the apples in a baking dish.

4. In a small bowl, mix together the butter, brown sugar, and cinnamon.

5. Spoon the butter mixture into the center of each apple.

6. If using walnuts, sprinkle them over the top of the butter mixture.

7. Bake the apples for 25-30 minutes, or until they are tender and the filling is golden brown.

8. Serve the apples hot and enjoy!

Prep Time: 10 minutes

Cook Time: 25-30 minutes

NUTRITIONAL VALUE **(per serving):**

Calories: 205; Fat: 10g; Carbohydrates: 31g; Fiber: 5g; Sugar: 24g; Protein: 1g.

These Baked Apples are a healthy and delicious dessert that's perfect for satisfying your sweet tooth. The butter, brown sugar, and cinnamon fillinaddds a warm and comforting flavor, while the nuts give a nice crunch and added nutrition. Plus, this recipe is easy to customize by using different types of apples or adding your favorite toppings. Give it a try and enjoy this simple yet satisfying dessert!

4. CHOCOLATE CHIA PUDDING RECIPE

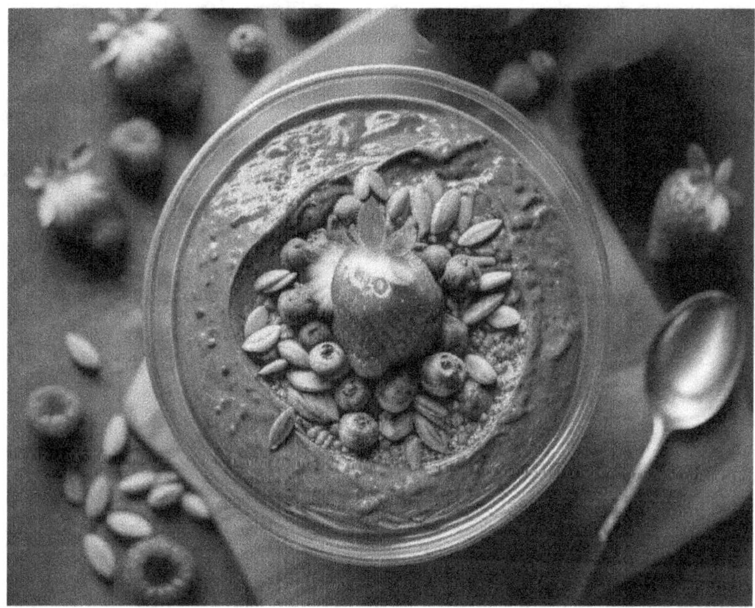

This Chocolate Chia Pudding is a healthy and delicious dessert that's perfect for satisfying your sweet tooth. It's packed with protein, fiber, and essential nutrients, and it's easy to make with just a few simple ingredients.

INGREDIENTS:

- 1/4 cup chia seeds

- 1 cup almond milk (or milk of your choice)

- 2 tbsp cocoa powder

- 2 tbsp maple syrup (or sweetener of your choice)

- 1/2 tsp vanilla extract

- Pinch of salt

- Optional toppings: chopped nuts, coconut flakes, fresh berries

1. In a bowl, whisk together the chia seeds, almond milk, cocoa powder, maple syrup, vanilla extract, and salt until well combined.

2. Cover the bowl and place it in the fridge for at least 2-3 hours, or overnight, until the chia pudding has thickened and the seeds have absorbed the liquid.

3. Once the chia pudding is ready, stir it well to make sure there are no clumps.

4. Divide the pudding into individual serving bowls or jars.

5. Tops with your favorite toppings, such as chopped nuts, coconut flakes, or fresh berries.

6. Serve and enjoy!

Prep Time: 5 minutes

Cook Time: 2-3 hours (or overnight)

NUTRITIONAL VALUE **(per serving):**

Calories: 232; Fat: 11g; Carbohydrates: 29g; Fiber: 12g; Sugar: 12g; Protein: 7g.

This Chocolate Chia Pudding is a healthier alternative to traditional chocolate pudding, and it's just as tasty and satisfying. The chia seeds provide protein, fiber, and essential omega-3 fatty acids, while the cocoa powder adds a rich chocolate flavor. Plus, this recipe is easy to customize by adding your favorite toppings. Give it a try and enjoy this guilt-free dessert!

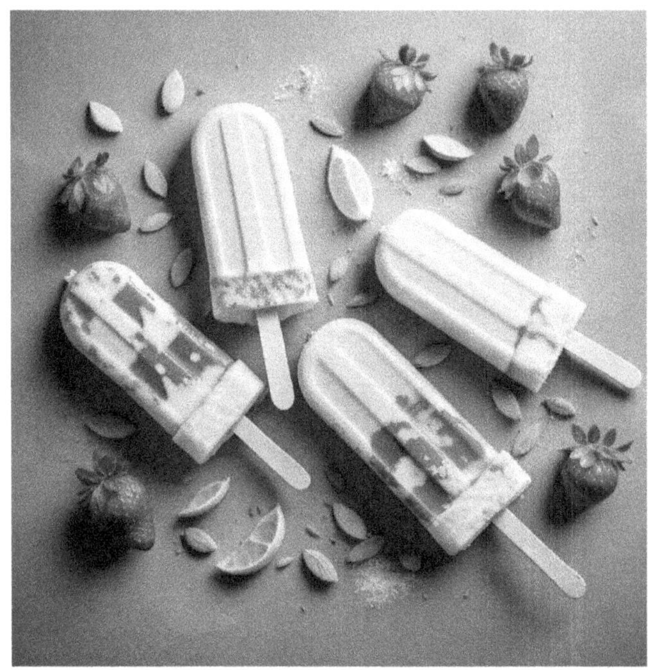

Looking for a healthy and refreshing treat to beat the summer heat? These Banana and Yogurt Popsicles are the perfect solution! They're easy to make, packed with nutrients, and they taste delicious.

INGREDIENTS:

- 2 ripe bananas

- 1 cup plain Greek yogurt

- 2 tbsp honey (or sweetener of your choice)

- 1 tsp vanilla extract

- Pinch of salt

COOKING INSTRUCTIONS:

1. Peel the bananas and place them in a blender.

2. Add the Greek yogurt, honey, vanilla extract, and salt to the blender.

3. Blend the mixture until smooth and creamy.

4. Pour the mixture into popsicle molds.

5. Place the molds in the freezer and let them freeze for at least 3-4 hours, or overnight.

6. Once the popsicles are frozen, remove them from the molds and enjoy!

Prep Time: 10 minutes

Freezing Time: 3-4 hours (or overnight)

NUTRITIONAL VALUE **(per serving):**

Calories: 95; Fat: 1g; Carbohydrates: 20g; Fiber: 1g; Sugar: 14g; Protein: 5g.

These Banana and Yogurt Popsicles are a healthy and delicious treat that's perfect for cooling down on a hot summer day. The bananas provide natural sweetness and essential nutrients like potassium, while the Greek yogurt adds protein and probiotics for a healthy gut. Plus, this recipe is easy to customize by adding your favorite fruits or toppings. Give it a try and enjoy a guilt-free dessert!

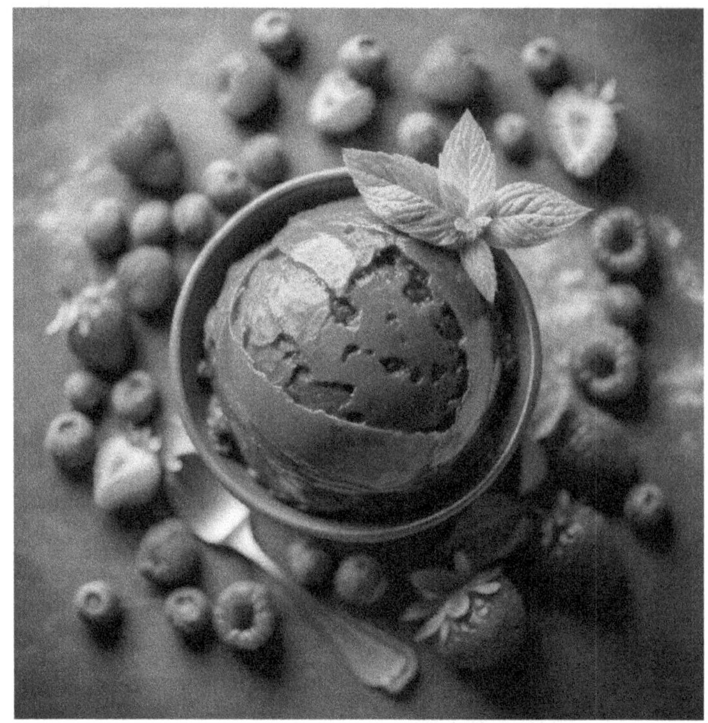

This Mixed Berry Sorbet is a refreshing and healthy dessert that's perfect for summertime. It's made with a variety of fresh berries, and it's easy to make with just a few simple ingredients.

INGREDIENTS:

- 4 cups mixed berries (such as strawberries, raspberries, and blueberries)

- 1/2 cup water

- 1/2 cup honey (or sweetener of your choice)

- Juice of 1 lemon

COOKING INSTRUCTIONS:

1. Rinse and hull the strawberries.

2. Add the mixed berries, water, honey, and lemon juice to a blender.

3. Blend the mixture until smooth.

4. Pour the mixture into a container and place it in the freezer for at least 2-3 hours.

5. Once the mixture starts to freeze, remove it from the freezer and stir it to break up any ice crystals.

6. Place the mixture back in the freezer and repeat the process every 30-60 minutes until it has reached the desired consistency.

7. Once the sorbet is fully frozen, scoop it into serving bowls and enjoy!

Prep Time: 15 minutes

Freezing Time: 2-3 hours

NUTRITIONAL VALUE **(per serving):**

Calories: 106; Fat: 0g; Carbohydrates: 27g; Fiber: 3g; Sugar: 23g; Protein: 1g.

This Mixed Berry Sorbet is a healthy and refreshing dessert that's perfect for those hot summer days. The combination of fresh berries provides essential nutrients like vitamin C and antioxidants, while the honey adds natural sweetness. Plus, this recipe is easy to customize by using your favorite berries or adding a splash of coconut milk for a creamier texture. Give it a try and enjoy a guilt-free treat!

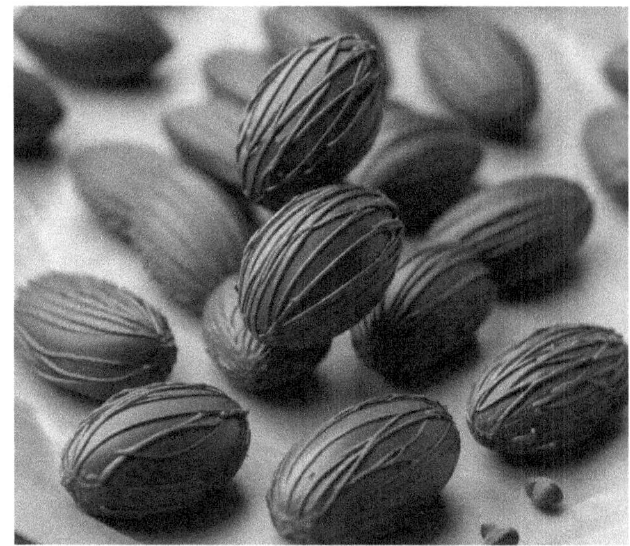

These Dark Chocolate Covered Almonds are a delicious and healthier alternative to traditional candy. They're easy to make, packed with nutrients, and they taste great!

INGREDIENTS:

- 1 cup raw almonds

- 8 oz. dark chocolate chips or chopped dark chocolate

- Sea salt (optional)

COOKING INSTRUCTIONS:

1. Preheat the oven to 350°F.

2. Spread the raw almonds on a baking sheet and roast for 10-15 minutes, or until lightly toasted.

3. Remove the almonds from the oven and let them cool for a few minutes.

4. While the almonds are cooling, melt the dark chocolate in a double boiler or a microwave-safe bowl. Stir the chocolate frequently until it's completely melted and smooth.

5. Add the roasted almonds to the melted chocolate and stir until they're fully coated.

6. Use a slotted spoon to remove the chocolate-covered almonds from the bowl and place them onto a baking sheet lined with parchment paper.

7. Sprinkle a pinch of sea salt over the chocolate-covered almonds (optional).

8. Place the baking sheet in the refrigerator for 1 hour, or until the chocolate is firm.

9. Once the chocolate is firm, remove the almonds from the baking sheet and store them in an airtight container.

Prep Time: 10 minutes

Cooking Time: 15 minutes

Chilling Time: 1 hour

NUTRITIONAL VALUE **(per serving):**

Calories: 216; Fat: 15g; Carbohydrates: 16g; Fiber: 4g; Sugar: 10g; Protein: 5g.

These Dark Chocolate Covered Almonds are a healthy and delicious snack that's perfect for satisfying your sweet tooth. The almonds provide fiber, protein, and healthy fats, while the dark chocolate adds antioxidants and a rich flavor. Plus, this recipe is easy to customize by adding your favorite toppings like shredded coconut or chopped nuts. Give it a try and enjoy a guilt-free treat!

BEVERAGES

A. FRUIT-INFUSED WATER

Staying hydrated during pregnancy is crucial, but drinking plain water can get boring after a while. Fruit-infused water is a tasty and refreshing alternative that is packed with flavor and nutrients. Here are three simple and delicious recipes for fruit-infused water that are perfect for pregnant women:

1. LEMON AND GINGER DETOX WATER

- 1 lemon, sliced

- 1-inch ginger root, peeled and sliced

- 4 cups water

Combine all ingredients in a pitcher and let sit in the fridge for at least one hour (or overnight) before drinking.

2. STRAWBERRY AND MINT WATER

- 1 cup strawberries, hulled and sliced

- 5-6 mint leaves

- 4 cups water

Combine all ingredients in a pitcher and let sit in the fridge for at least one hour (or overnight) before drinking.

3. CUCUMBER AND LIME WATER

- 1/2 cucumber, sliced

- 1 lime, sliced

- 4 cups water

Combine all ingredients in a pitcher and let sit in the fridge for at least one hour (or overnight) before drinking.

These fruit-infused water recipes are a healthy and tasty way to stay hydrated during pregnancy. They are packed with vitamins, minerals, and antioxidants, and are a great alternative to sugary drinks. Plus, they are easy to make and can be customized with your favorite fruits and herbs.

B. HERBAL TEA BLENDS FOR PREGNANCY

Drinking herbal teas during pregnancy can provide many benefits such as easing pregnancy-related symptoms and improving overall health. However, it is important to choose teas that are safe for pregnancy and avoid those that may cause harm. Here are three herbal tea blends that are considered safe and beneficial for pregnant women:

1. GINGER TEA

Ginger has anti-inflammatory and anti-nausea properties and can be helpful in alleviating morning sickness and nausea during pregnancy. To make ginger tea, steep 1-2 teaspoons of freshly grated ginger in hot water for 5-10 minutes. Honey or lemon can be added for flavor.

2. RED RASPBERRY LEAF TEA

Red raspberry leaf tea contains high levels of vitamins, minerals, and antioxidants and is known to strengthen the uterus in preparation for labor. It is recommended to start drinking red raspberry leaf tea in the second trimester. To make the tea, steep 1-2 teaspoons of dried red raspberry leaf in hot water for 5-10 minutes.

3. PEPPERMINT TEA

Peppermint tea can help relieve digestive issues such as bloating, gas, and nausea, which are common during pregnancy. It can also help reduce stress and improve mental clarity. To make peppermint tea, steep 1-2 teaspoons of dried peppermint leaves in hot water for 5-10 minutes.

It is important to note that pregnant women should limit their caffeine intake to 200 mg per day, which is roughly the amount in one 12-ounce cup of coffee. It is also important to consult with a healthcare provider before adding any herbal teas or supplements to your diet during pregnancy.

4. CHAMOMILE TEA

Chamomile tea is a natural relaxant, which can help reduce stress and promote better sleep during pregnancy. It can also help alleviate digestive discomfort and reduce inflammation. To make chamomile tea, steep 1-2 teaspoons of dried chamomile flowers in hot water for 5-10 minutes.

5. LEMON BALM TEA

Lemon balm tea contains antioxidants and has calming properties that can help reduce anxiety and promote relaxation during pregnancy. It can also help alleviate digestive issues and promote better sleep. To make lemon balm tea, steep 1-2 teaspoons of dried lemon balm leaves in hot water for 5-10 minutes.

As always, it is important to consult with a healthcare provider before adding any herbal teas or supplements to your diet during pregnancy.

HEALTHY AND DELICIOUS SMOOTHIES

Smoothies can be a great way to pack in lots of healthy nutrients in one delicious drink!

Here are two recipes for healthy and delicious smoothies:

1. GREEN SMOOTHIE:

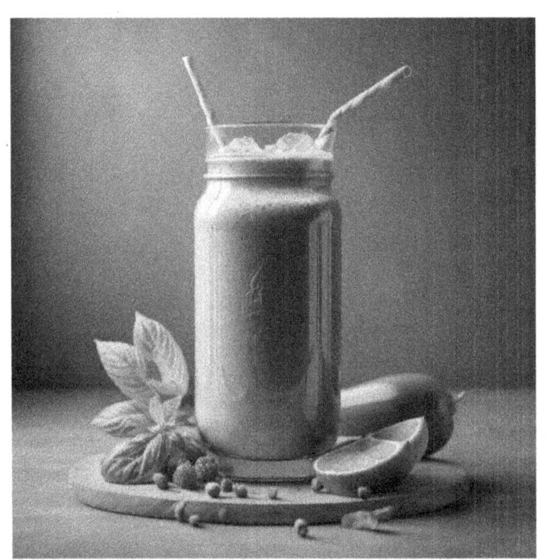

INGREDIENTS:

- 1 banana, sliced

- 2 cups spinach

- 1 celery stalk, chopped

- 1 tbsp chia seeds

- 1 cup unsweetened almond milk

- 1 tsp honey (optional)

1. Add all ingredients to a blender and blend until smooth.

2. Pour into a glass and enjoy!

This smoothie is packed with vitamins and minerals from spinach and celery, and the chia seeds provide healthy omega-3 fats. The banana adds natural sweetness and the almond milk gives the smoothie a creamy texture.

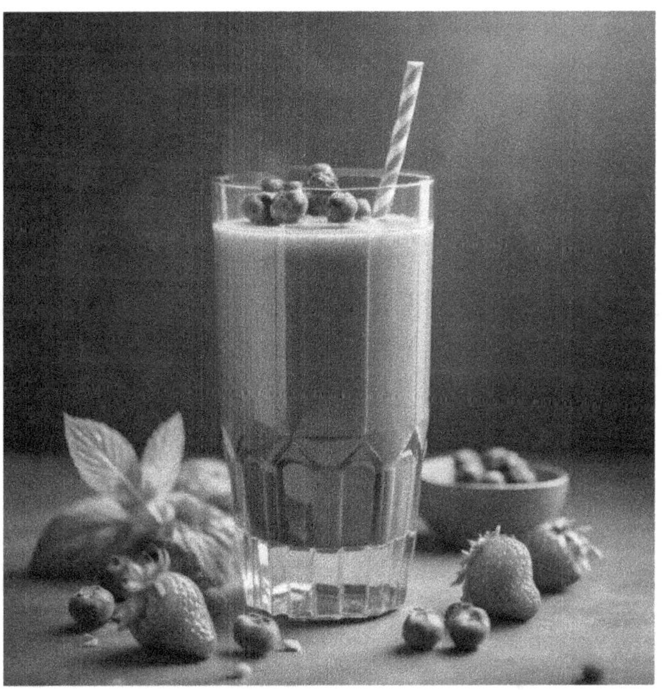

- 1 cup mixed berries (strawberries, blueberries, raspberries)

- 1 banana

- 1 cup unsweetened almond milk

- 1 tbsp almond butter

- 1 tsp honey (optional)

1. Add all ingredients to a blender and blend until smooth.

2. Pour into a glass and enjoy!

This smoothie is loaded with antioxidants from the berries, and the almond butter provides healthy fats and protein. The banana adds natural sweetness and the almond milk gives the smoothie a creamy texture.

3. TROPICAL SMOOTHIE

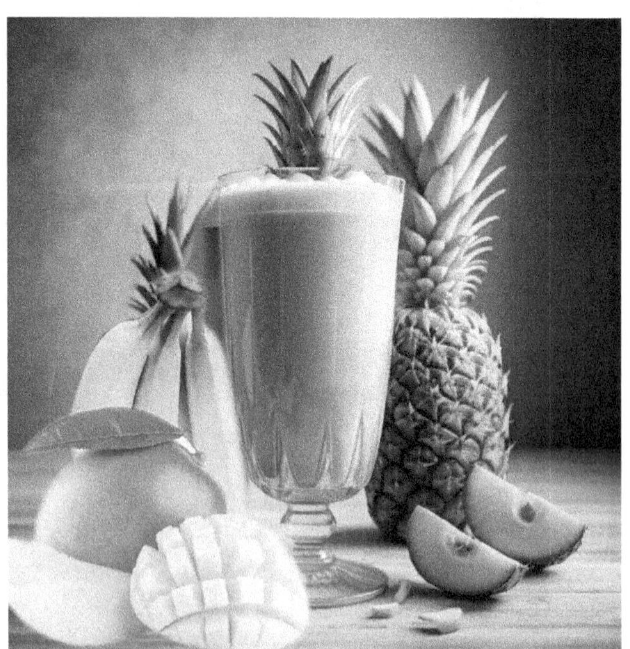

INGREDIENTS:

- 1 cup frozen pineapple chunks

- 1 cup frozen mango chunks

- 1 banana

- 1 cup unsweetened coconut milk

- 1 tsp grated fresh ginger

DIRECTIONS:

1. Add all ingredients to a blender and blend until smooth.

2. Pour into a glass and enjoy!

This smoothie is rich in vitamin C, fiber, and essential minerals, and ginger can help alleviate nausea and reduce inflammation during pregnancy.

4. BLUEBERRY YOGURT SMOOTHIE

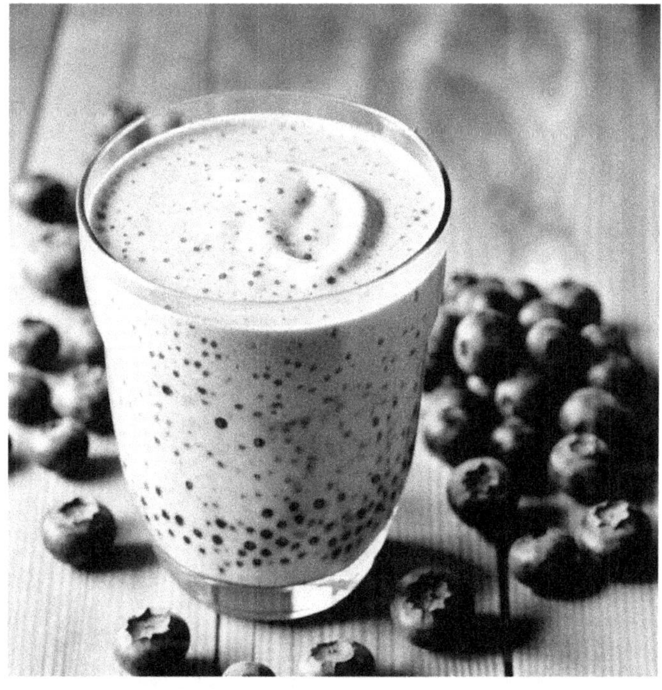

- 1 cup frozen blueberries

- 1 cup plain Greek yogurt

- 1 banana

- 1 tbsp honey

- 1 tsp vanilla extract

- 1 cup almond milk

DIRECTIONS:

1. Add all ingredients to a blender and blend until smooth.

2. Pour into a glass and enjoy!

This smoothie is packed with protein from the Greek yogurt, and the blueberries provide antioxidants and anti-inflammatory compounds that can benefit both mom and baby during pregnancy.

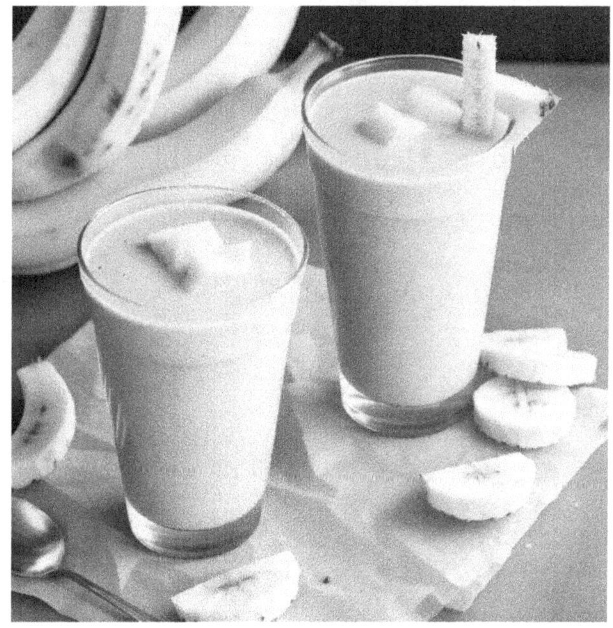

INGREDIENTS:

- 1 banana

- 1 tbsp peanut butter

- 1 cup unsweetened almond milk

- 1 tsp honey

- 1 tsp cinnamon

DIRECTIONS:

1. Add all ingredients to a blender and blend until smooth.

2. Pour into a glass and enjoy!

This smoothie is high in protein, healthy fats, and fiber, making it a great pick-me-up during pregnancy. Cinnamon can also help regulate blood sugar levels and reduce cravings.

Remember to use fresh or frozen fruits and vegetables, and use a high-speed blender for the best results. You can also customize these recipes to your liking by adding or substituting ingredients as you see fit. Enjoy!

CHAPTER 8

CONCLUSION

RECAP OF THE HEALTH BENEFITS OF A PREGNANCY-FRIENDLY DIET

A pregnancy-friendly diet is essential to support the growth and development of your baby, as well as to maintain your own health during pregnancy. By following a balanced diet that includes high-quality proteins, healthy fats, and a variety of fruits and vegetables, you can give your baby the nutrients they need to grow and thrive. Some of the health benefits of a pregnancy-friendly diet include:

1. Optimal fetal development: A diet rich in essential nutrients like folic acid, iron, and calcium can support your baby's growth and development, from the early stages of pregnancy through birth.

2. Reduced risk of complications: Studies have shown that mothers who follow a healthy diet during pregnancy have a lower risk of developing gestational diabetes, high blood pressure, and other complications.

3. Improved mood and energy: Eating a well-balanced diet can help improve your energy levels and reduce mood swings, both of which are common during pregnancy.

4. Support for breastfeeding: A healthy pregnancy diet can lay the foundation for good nutrition while breastfeeding, providing the nutrients your baby needs to grow and develop.

In short, a pregnancy-friendly diet is crucial for maintaining your health and promoting the optimal growth and development of your baby. By making smart choices and prioritizing nutrient-dense foods, you can set yourself and your baby up for a healthy, happy pregnancy and beyond.

ADDITIONAL TIPS FOR MAINTAINING A HEALTHY LIFESTYLE DURING PREGNANCY

In addition to following a healthy pregnancy diet, there are several other tips that can help you maintain a healthy lifestyle during pregnancy. These include:

1. Staying active: Regular exercise during pregnancy can help boost your energy, reduce stress, and even make labor and delivery easier. Talk to your healthcare provider about safe exercise options and aim for at least 30 minutes of activity most days of the week.

2. Getting enough rest: Pregnancy can be exhausting, so be sure to prioritize rest and relaxation. Aim for 7-9 hours of sleep each night and take naps or breaks throughout the day as needed.

3. Managing stress: Pregnancy can be a stressful time, so it's important to find healthy ways to manage stress. Try techniques like meditation, deep breathing, or prenatal yoga to help you relax.

4. Drinking enough water: Staying hydrated is crucial for both you and your baby. Aim for at least 8 glasses of water per day and pay attention to your thirst cues.

5. Avoiding harmful substances: This includes smoking, alcohol, and certain medications or substances that can be harmful to your baby. Talk to your healthcare provider about any medications you're taking to ensure they're safe during pregnancy.

By following these additional tips, you can help ensure a safe and healthy pregnancy for you and your baby. Consulting with your healthcare provider and making healthy choices in all aspects of your life will help to pave the way for a successful pregnancy, childbirth, and postpartum experience.

Encouragement for readers to try new recipes and embrace healthy eating

In conclusion, a healthy pregnancy diet is essential for both you and your baby. However, healthy eating doesn't have to be boring or tasteless. Don't be afraid to experiment with new recipes or modify the ones in this book to suit your taste preferences. By making healthy eating fun and enjoyable, you'll be more likely to stick with it throughout your pregnancy and beyond. Remember, every healthy choice you make is a step towards a healthy pregnancy and a healthy baby.

So, don't hesitate to try new things, get creative, and enjoy the journey towards a healthy lifestyle. You got this!

As an author, I believe that feedback from my readers is crucial in improving my writing and providing a better experience for future readers. Therefore, I would like to request sincere feedback from those who have read this book.

I would appreciate it if you could share your honest thoughts and opinions about the book. What did you like about it? What could I have done better? Did it provide new insights? Did it help you in any way?

Your honest feedback will help me improve and provide an even better experience for readers in the future. Please feel free to share your opinions, suggestions, and criticisms.

Thank you for taking the time to read and provide your feedback. Your support and input are invaluable, and I look forward to hearing from you.